Sod and Chlory

The adventurous journey of a salt crystal

through the depths of our body

1st Edition

March 22, 2022

Impressum

Text + Images: © Copyright 2022
Hans Oberleithner
6065 Thaur
Austria

Dedicated to

(in chronological order)

Alva, Mattis, Kassian, Gabriel, Joscha & Lukas

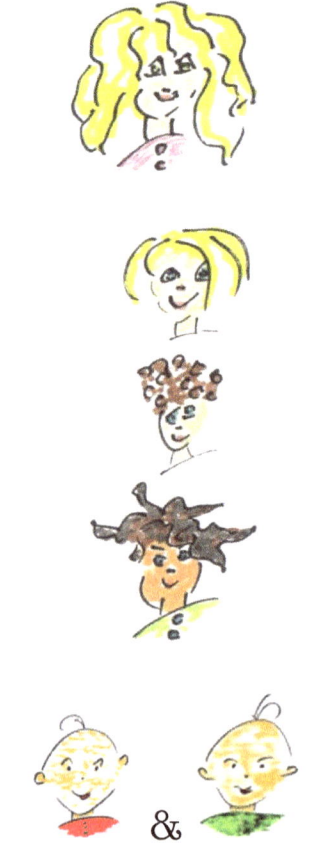

... and many others!

Contents

Sod and **Chlory** travel from the mountains to the sea..**4**

Sod and **Chlory** travel through mouth, stomach and intestine...**16**

Sod and **Chlory** travel through liver, heart and lung..**35**

Sod and **Chlory** travel through the head **45**

Sod and **Chlory** travel through spleen, kidney and bladder into the open..........................**55**

Sod and Chlory travel from the mountains to the sea

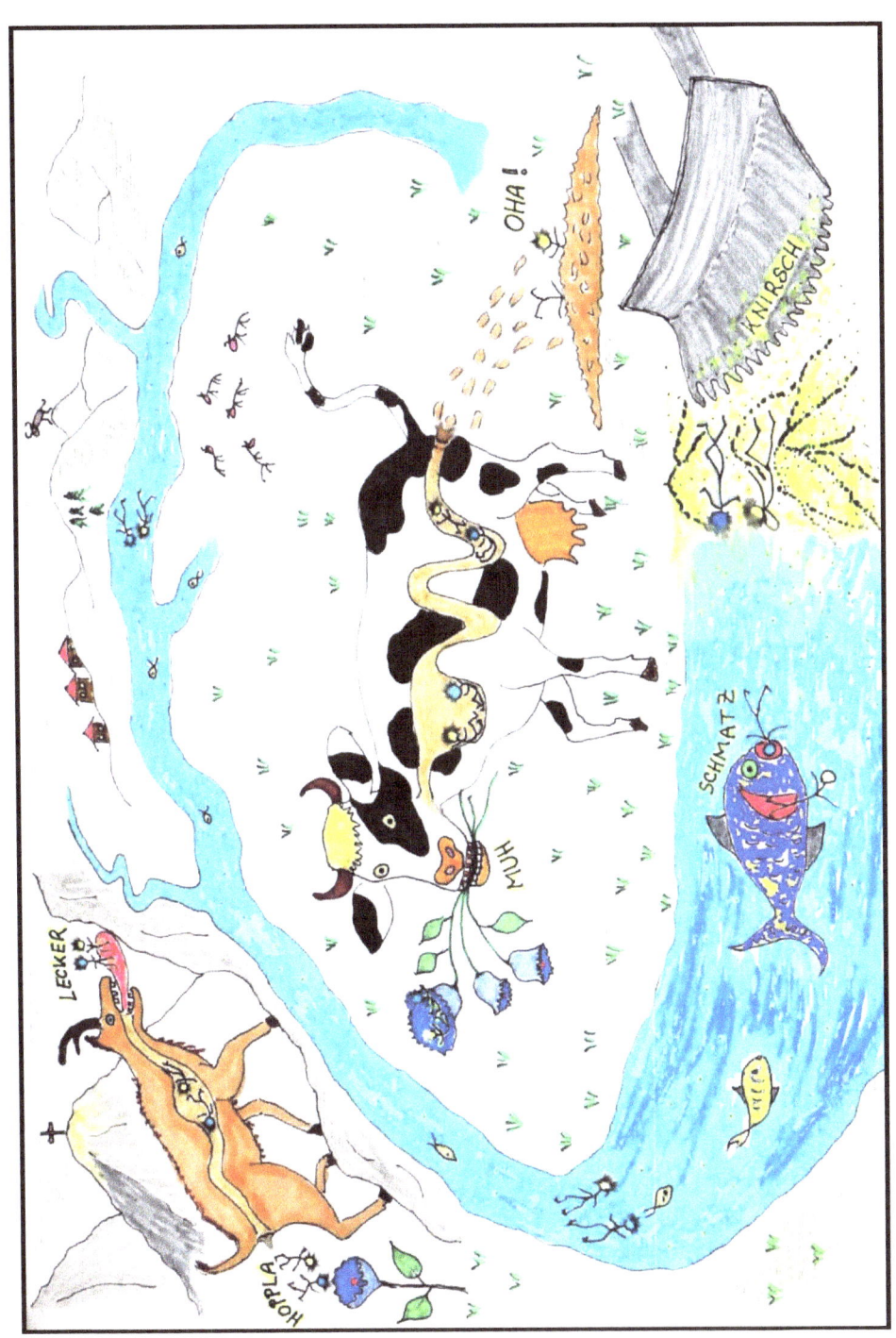

"**Chlory**," whispers **Sod**, "we're about to go?"

Chlory lolls over and squints through the glass into the sun. For quite some time now, the two have been sitting in a **salt shaker**.

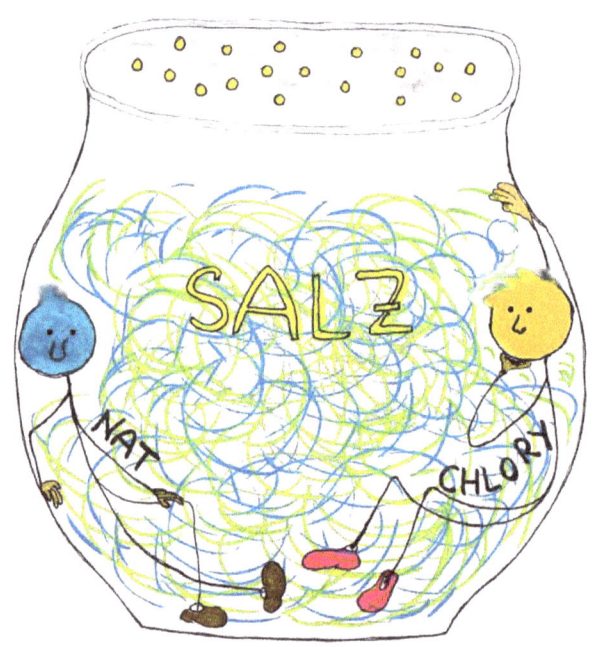

In the past, **Sod** and **Chlory** have traveled quite a bit. Ages ago, they had gotten stuck on the sticky tongue of a mountain chamois and then had gone through an exciting journey.

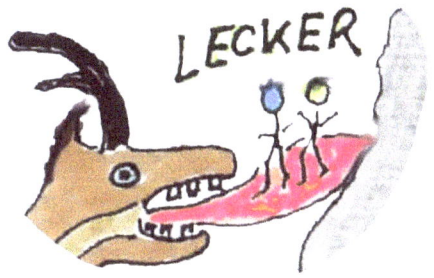

Because in the stomach of the chamois they came across a rare magic herb, that transformed them into tiny humans.
Suddenly they could

see,

hear,

speak,

cry and laugh

No more and no less.

Then they were dropped off by the chamois on a blooming alpine pasture.

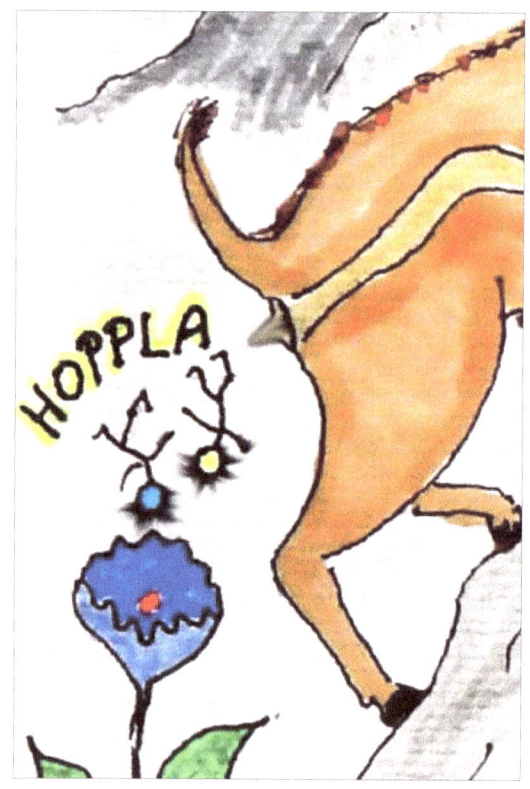

How long they lay there, in the soil between gentian, bluebells and blades of grass, that they don't know. For **Sod** and **Chlory**, it doesn't matter at all.

Why?

Because they do not age.
They are neither young nor old.
Together they form a grain of salt
that never fades.

On the alpine pasture, the two of them finally floated up in the stem of a bellflower, from the root to the blossom. No sooner had they made themselves comfortable in the blue flower calyx than they were being eaten by a black-spotted cow.

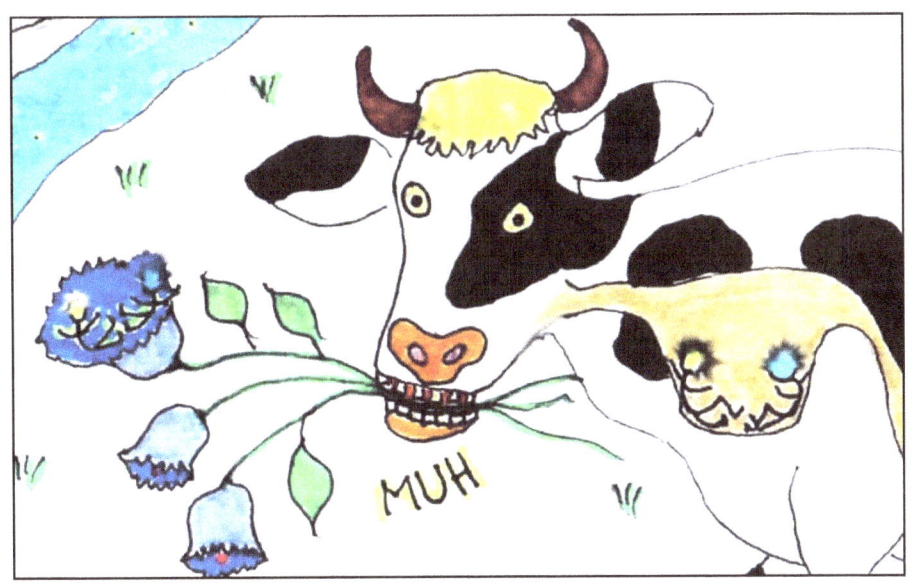

There they sat for a while in the cow's stomach and waited patiently until, after an exciting roller coaster ride through the cow's belly, they landed again on the alpine pasture, inside a steaming cow dung.

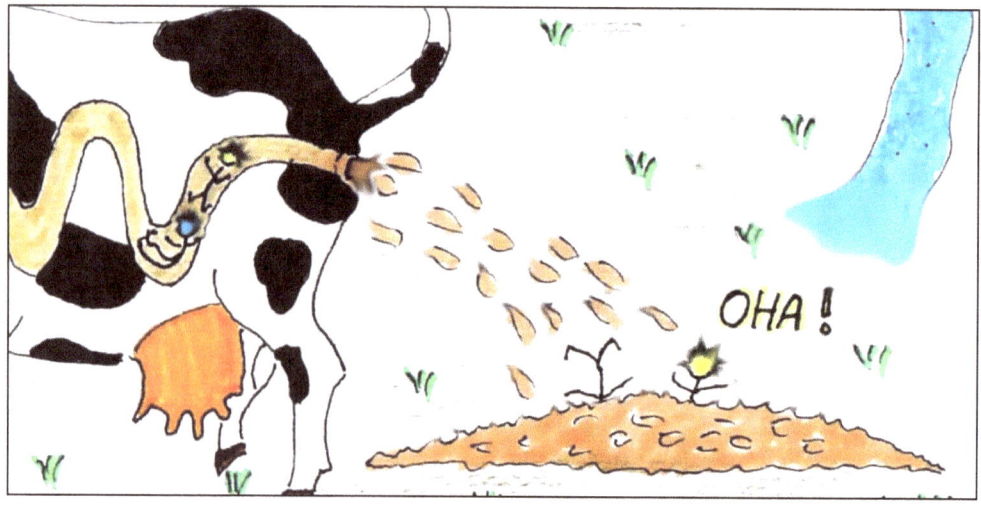

There, they spent the winter, and finally, in the spring, they were washed with the melt water down into the valley.

But that was only the beginning of a long journey.

A large river carried them over many weeks - it also could have been several years - all the way to the sea.

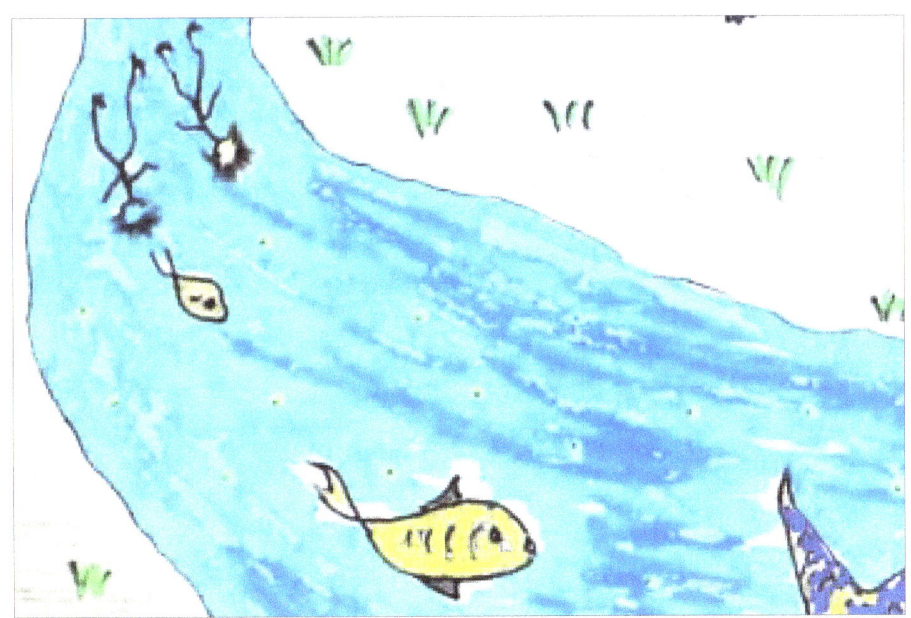

How scary was her first encounter with a fish that scooped them up in its giant mouth and immediately washed them back into the sea through its gills.

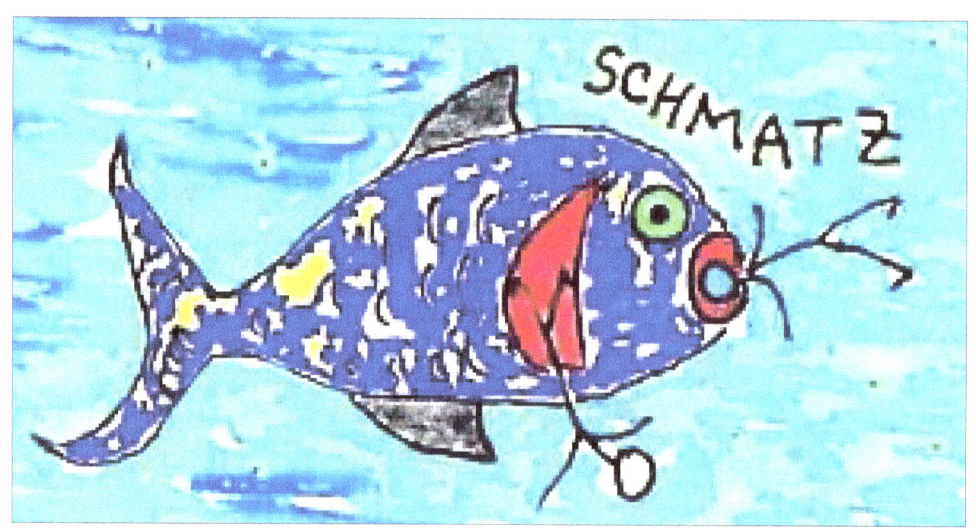

Fortunately, **Sod** is always near **Chlory**, so she never has to worry about losing him on these trips.

*Because **Sod** and **Chlory** are attracted*
to each other, like two magnets.
They always stay together, no matter what.

At some point, the two of them had been stranded on a beach and had let the sun dry them. More and more of their brothers and sisters, also glittering crystals, joined them until the beach was nothing but shiny salt. How they finally ended up in the salt shaker from there, that remains a mystery to them.

As **Sod** recalls, they were lying sparkling in the sun at the time just like every other morning.

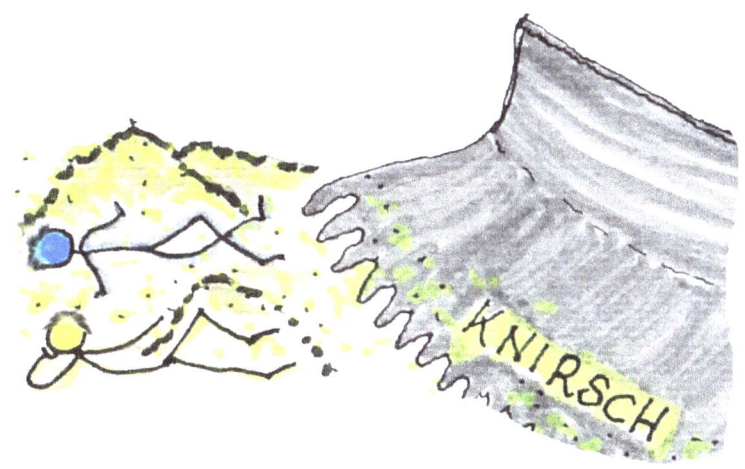

There he heard a crunching sound in a distance, gradually getting closer. Finally, he saw the shovel of an excavator coming toward him.

Sod pressed **Chlory** tightly against him, it whirled them around violently, and a little later they landed on a huge truck that took them rumbling away from the beach.

Neither **Sod** nor **Chlory** remember what happened after that. Maybe because it was too dark and they lost their orientation. Or because they simply slept for a long, long time. In any case, they woke up in a *salt shaker*, surrounded by their siblings who had traveled with them.

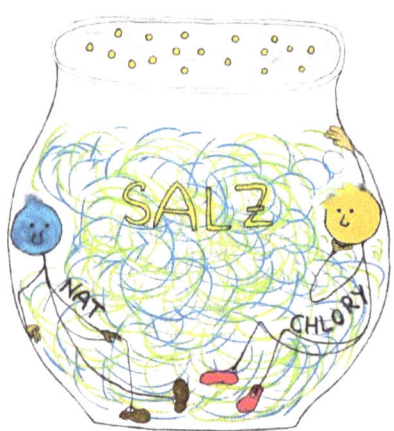

Thousands and thousands of sparkling crystals!

But now, they are at the beginning of a long journey.

While **Chlory** is still lolling around in the sun, motion pops up in the lively globetrotters. Amazed, they look out of the salt shaker, their little glass house. There, they see Moritz sitting at dinner, in front of a large plate of pasta.

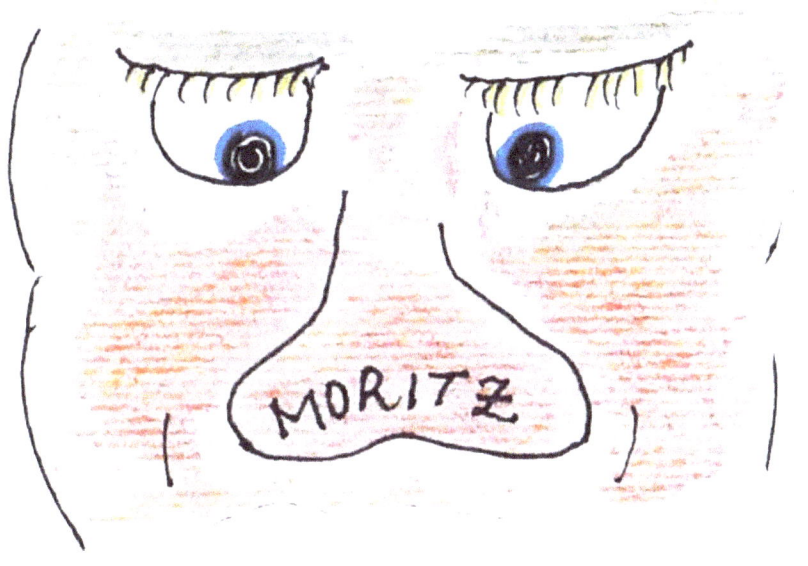

Sod and Chlory travel through mouth, stomach and intestine

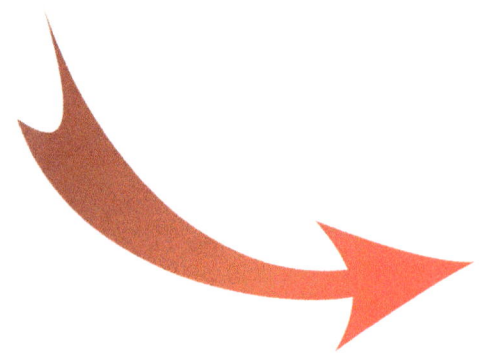

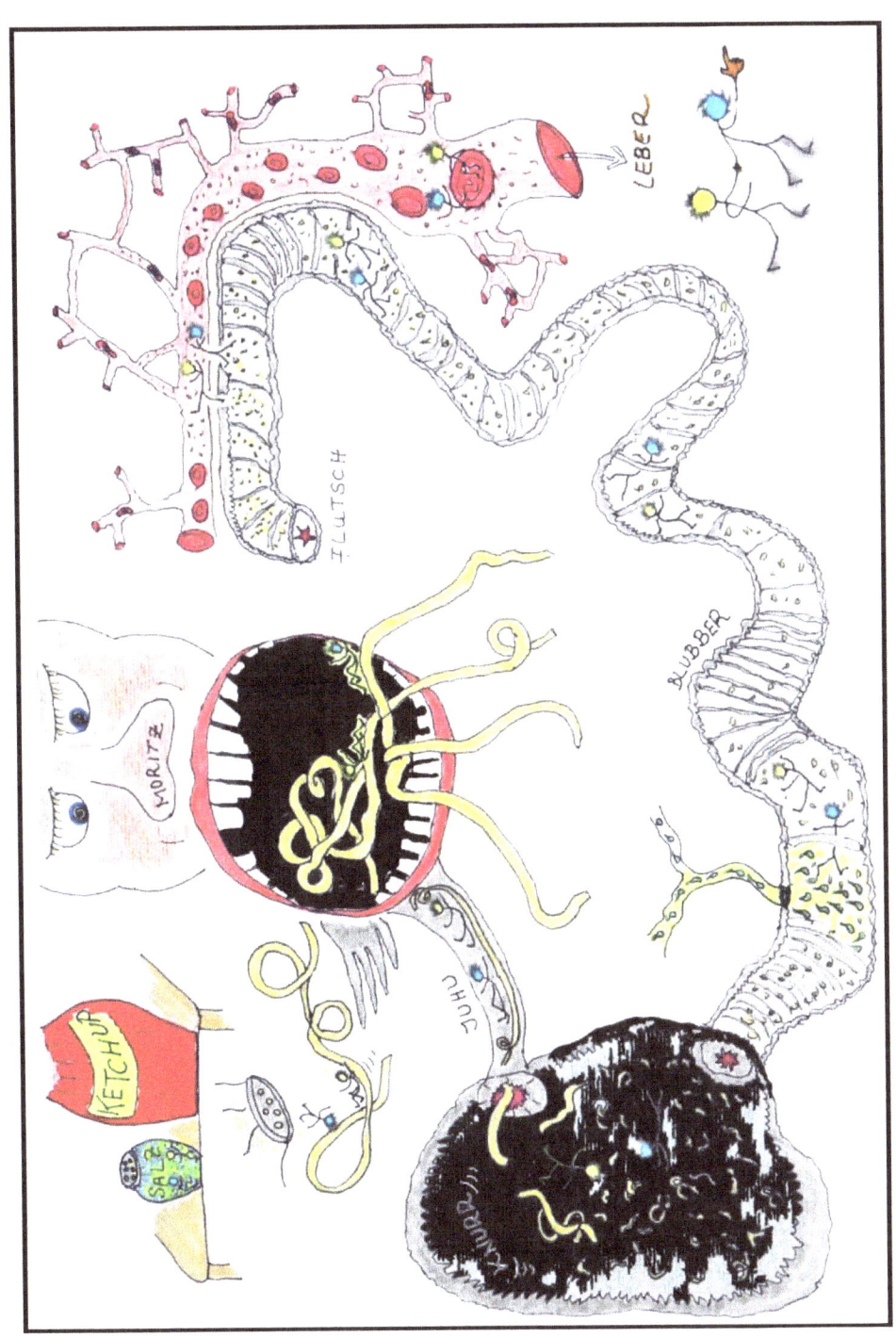

"**Chlory**, I think we're about to get our turn!" whispers **Sod**.

Sure enough, in the next moment their little glass house is lifted up, turned upside down, and **Sod** and **Chlory**, along with their siblings, are already trickling out through the holey roof.

"Where do you think we're going?" **Sod** calls out curiously, holding **Chlory** tightly so as not to lose her. Shortly after, they land softly on a trampoline, get tossed up a few times, and then settle down, exhausted.

"The trampoline is a spaghetti noodle, after all, and we're lying on it," **Chlory** says in amazement.

"**Watch out**, I see a fork coming at us right now, hold on tight!" yells **Sod**.

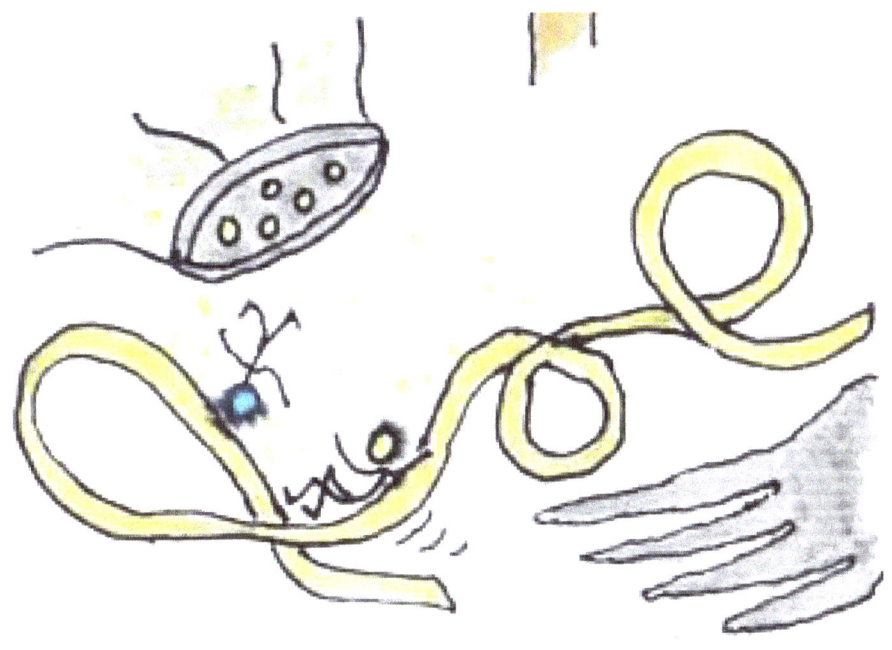

It's Moritz, now coiling a particularly long noodle, the very one on which **Sod** and **Chlory** are stretched out, around his fork.

"I'm almost getting dizzy," **Chlory** shrieks delightedly, for she loves the airstream.

Sod crawls to the surface, **Chlory** in tow.

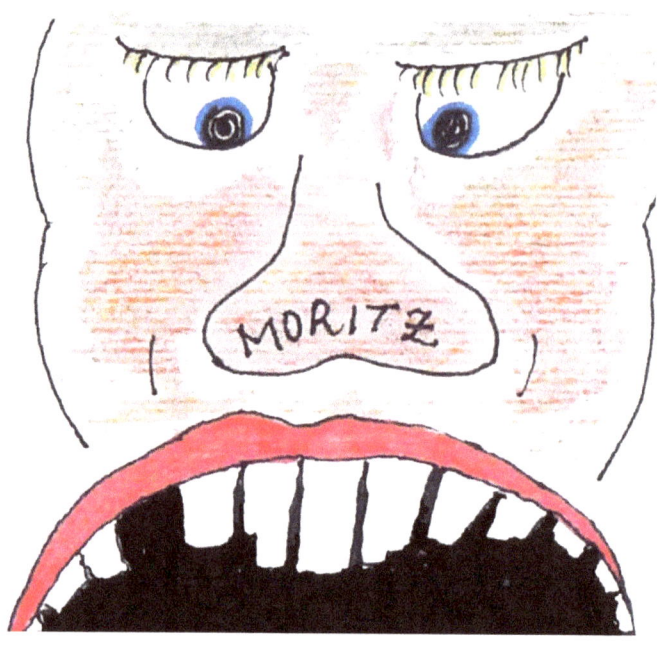

Suddenly, fear grips them.

A gate opens up in front of them.
"Reminds me of a fish mouth, like we saw in the sea that time," **Chlory** whispers, having recovered from the initial shock. "I wonder if we'll get flushed back out there, too?" murmurs **Sod** thoughtfully. But they can't think about it for

long, because the noodle is already disappearing into the darkness along with them.

"Have we landed in a cave here?" asks **Chlory** somewhat despondently, thinking wistfully of the sunny beach by the sea.

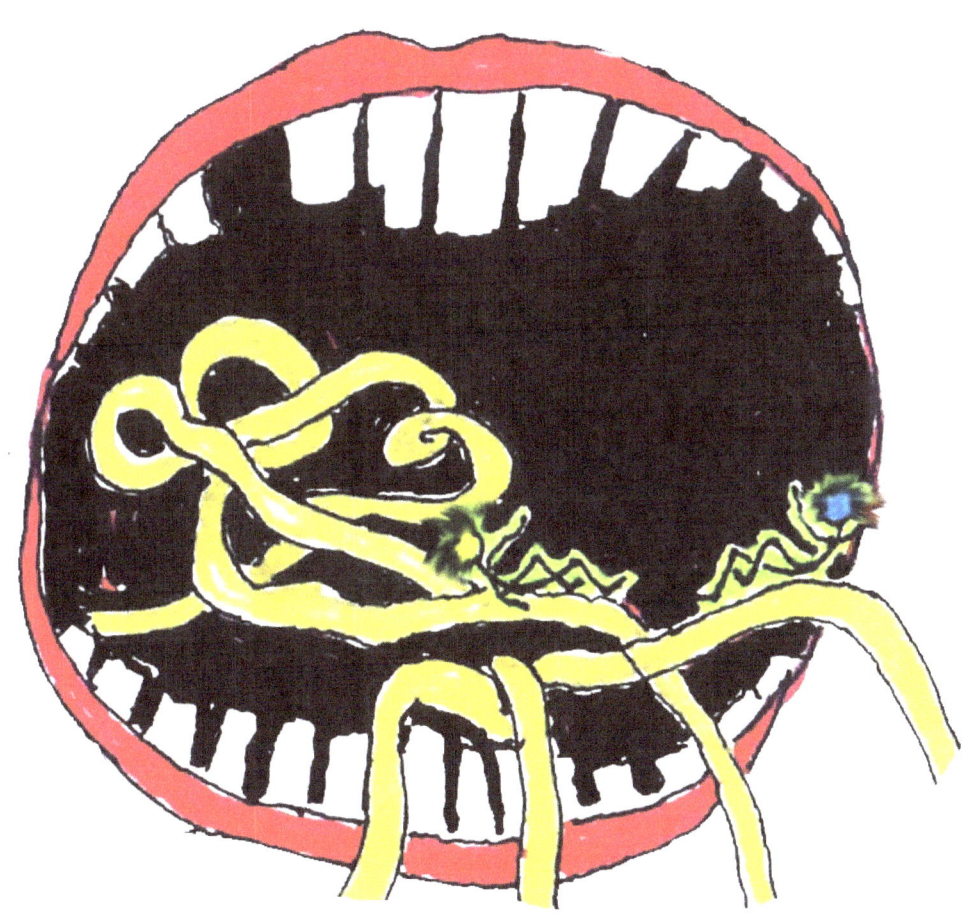

"Pretty damp in here," **Sod** observes.

"No wonder, with torrents flowing down from the walls," **Chlory** adds quietly.

Again and again, the Moritz gate opens and more noodles jump off the fork. Like on a roller coaster, **Sod** and **Chlory** are being tossed around inside the cave.

Yes, indeed, they are in the middle of the mouth cavity of Moritz, who is having dinner. The two get to know every nook and cranny. Sometimes they stick to the top of the palate for a few seconds, then they climb a bit up the cheek to be dropped back onto the tongue with a loud splash.

Then **Sod** listens up, there's a deafening creak.

"I think we're about to get swallowed," he whispers in **Chlory's** ear.

Chlory is excited.

She remembers that time they were swallowed by the black-spotted cow.

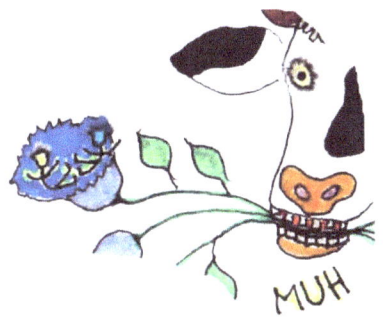

The cow's mouth was much roomier, she thinks, but admittedly it wasn't as soft there as it is today on the spaghetti noodle. Back then in the cow's mouth, they were whirled around between bulky grass stalks, so that after a while their crystal heads were really humming.

"Today is a special day, for the first time we are in a human mouth," **Chlory** says solemnly.
"We're about to go down the slide, through the esophagus straight into the stomach," **Sod** joy-

fully yells. With groans and creaks, the entrance door at the top of the slide opens. **Sod** and **Chlory** cling to their noodle.

"Do you remember, **Chlory**, how we used to watch the people on the surfboards by the sea? Now we surf like them too - down a slippery trail of slime into the dark maw!"

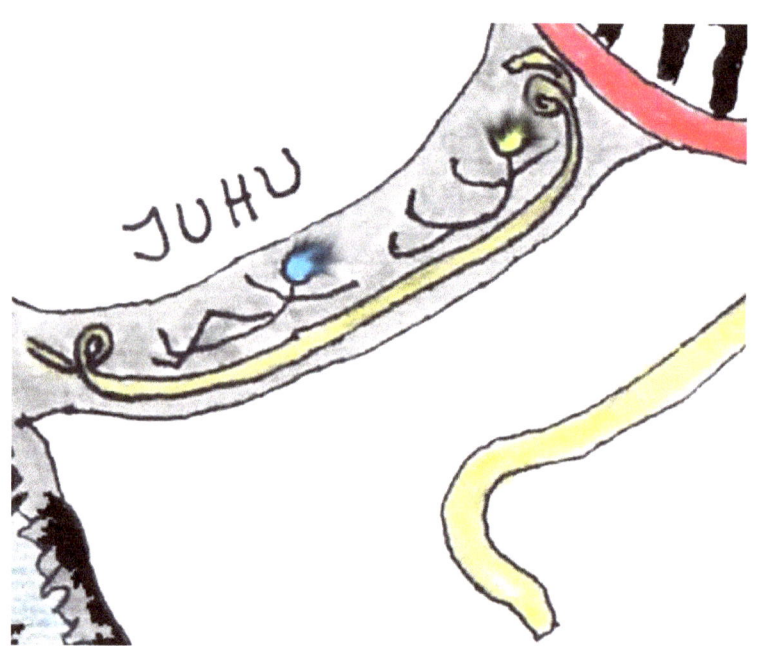

Chlory whoops as it starts.

The noodle is their surfboard, which they cling to. At one point, the noodle stops. Torrents of water shoot past them on the left and right, gurgling as they disappear into the darkness. But then it goes right on again.

Hooray! The noodle is the perfect surfboard!

Silky smooth, they slide with it to the end of the esophagus. It seems to be closed. **Sod** carefully straightens up so as not to fall off his surf noodle and knocks on a ring-shaped gate.

There's a creak and the ring widens around them.

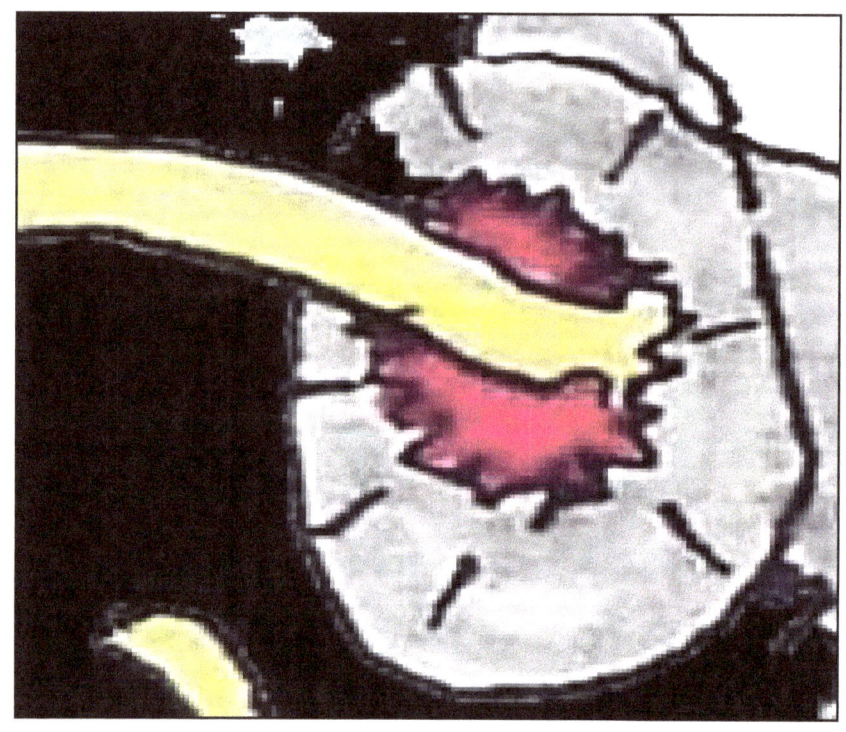

"We're standing at the entrance to the stomach!" exclaims **Sod** excitedly.

Suddenly, a loud growling can be heard from the depths.

The stomach has awakened and is writhing like a hungry dragon. Then her surf noodle receives a gentle nudge from behind and seconds later it glides elegantly into the stomach.

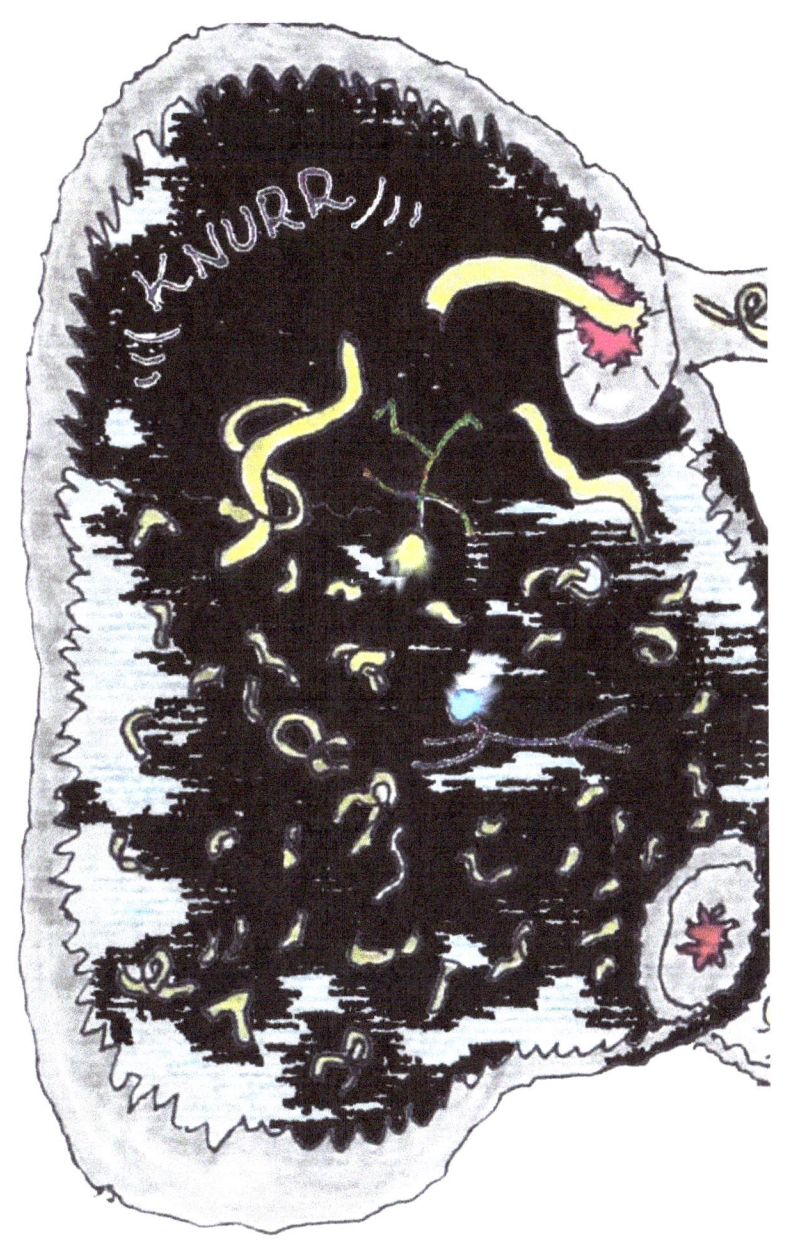

Inside the stomach there is a lot of hustle and bustle. New noodles constantly appear at the entrance to the stomach and plunge into the depths. Acid flows from deep crevices and chops up one noodle after another. Even **Sod** and **Chlory**'s surf noodle is not spared.

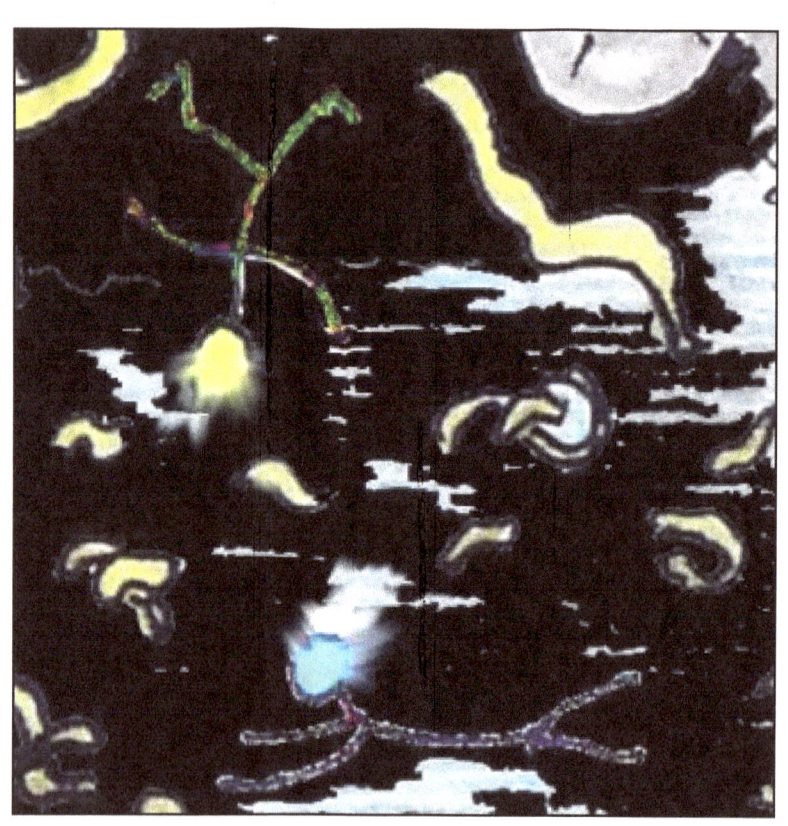

It slowly dissolves, so that the two have no choice but to plunge into the acidic waters. For

Sod and ***Chlory*** this is not bad, because their crystal body is invulnerable.

The two enjoy the refreshing bath in the stomach cavity. In he meantime, the spaghetti noodles have turned into a thick noodle mush that is getting closer and closer to the stomach exit. ***Sod*** sticks his head out of the noodle mush and knocks on the next ring-shaped gate that has appeared in front of them. It doesn't take long before it opens with a loud creak, revealing the way into a long winding tunnel. Majestically, the mash of noodles moves forward, with ***Sod*** and ***Chlory*** right in the middle of it.

"We've just entered the human bowel, I think," ***Sod*** exclaims eagerly.

"How would you know?" asks **Chlory** in amazement.

"Yes, I pricked up my ears when we were sitting in the salt shaker," says **Sod** gleefully, winking his eyes craftily.

"Because at dinner, I heard Moritz's *mother* say,

… Moritz don't put so many noodles in your mouth at once, or they'll get stuck in your esophagus or lie in your stomach like a big elephant that won't even fit in your intestines!"

In the intestine, it gets considerably tighter, but all the faster **Sod** and **Chlory** whiz around the first bend in their noodle mash.

"**Look out!**" shouts ***Chlory***, bravely swimming ahead. "There's a torrent coming in from the side, turning everything yellow".

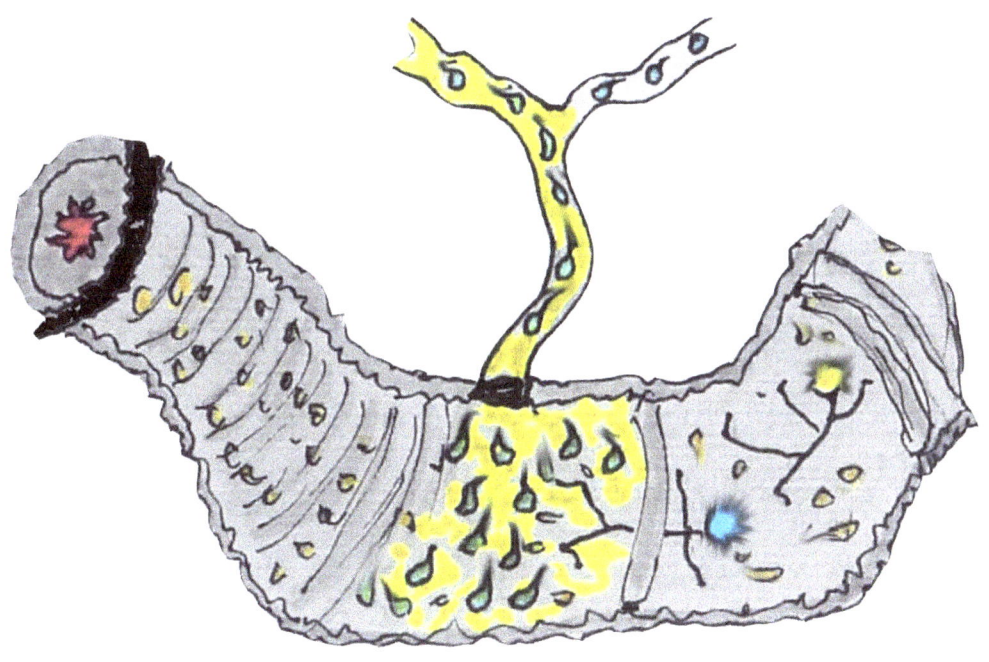

"Tastes pretty bitter," ***Sod*** adds, shivering. "Plus, I'm surrounded by hungry *greentails* that will eat anything that gets in their way".

"Just dive through," ***Chlory*** says, swimming bravely ahead.

After **Sod** and **Chlory** happily make it past the yellow fog zone with the voracious *greentails*, their journey continues amidst the noodle mash. They haven't encountered any surf noodles for a long time, because the *greentails* have smashed everything to bits. After some time, **Chlory** notices that the noodle mash is dwindling.

"If this keeps up, we'll soon be out on a limb," Glory thinks aloud. "**Sod**, do you have any idea where the noodle mush is vanishing to?"

"I think it just travels through the intestinal wall, right into Moritz," **Sod** says meaningfully, scratching his crystal head.

"But we're already inside Moritz," **Chlory** replies incredulously.

"Yes, we're in his gut, but we're not in his blood yet," **Sod** says promisingly. "Watch out, **Chlory**, we'll just hide in the pasta mush and at the first opportunity we'll migrate with the mush through the intestinal wall".

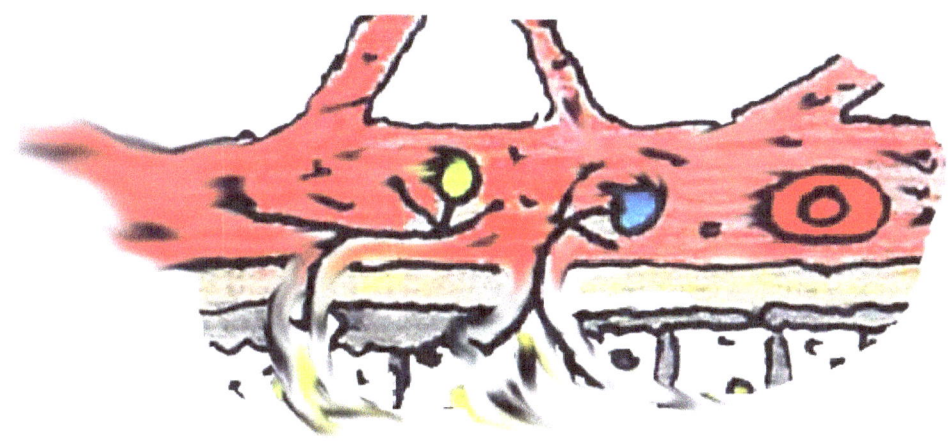

So **Sod** and **Chlory** swim up close to the intestinal wall. As soon as **Sod** touches the slippery wall, a tiny window opens and he slips through. **Chlory** also finds a window, right next to him, through which she can slip.
With a loud splash, they both land side by side in the blood that flows sluggishly past the out-

side of the intestinal wall. There are no more noodles to hold on to, but the place is teeming with little fiery red boats that whiz merrily past them. The two sit down in one of them and wait anxiously to see where the journey will take them.

Sod and Chlory travel through liver, heart and lung

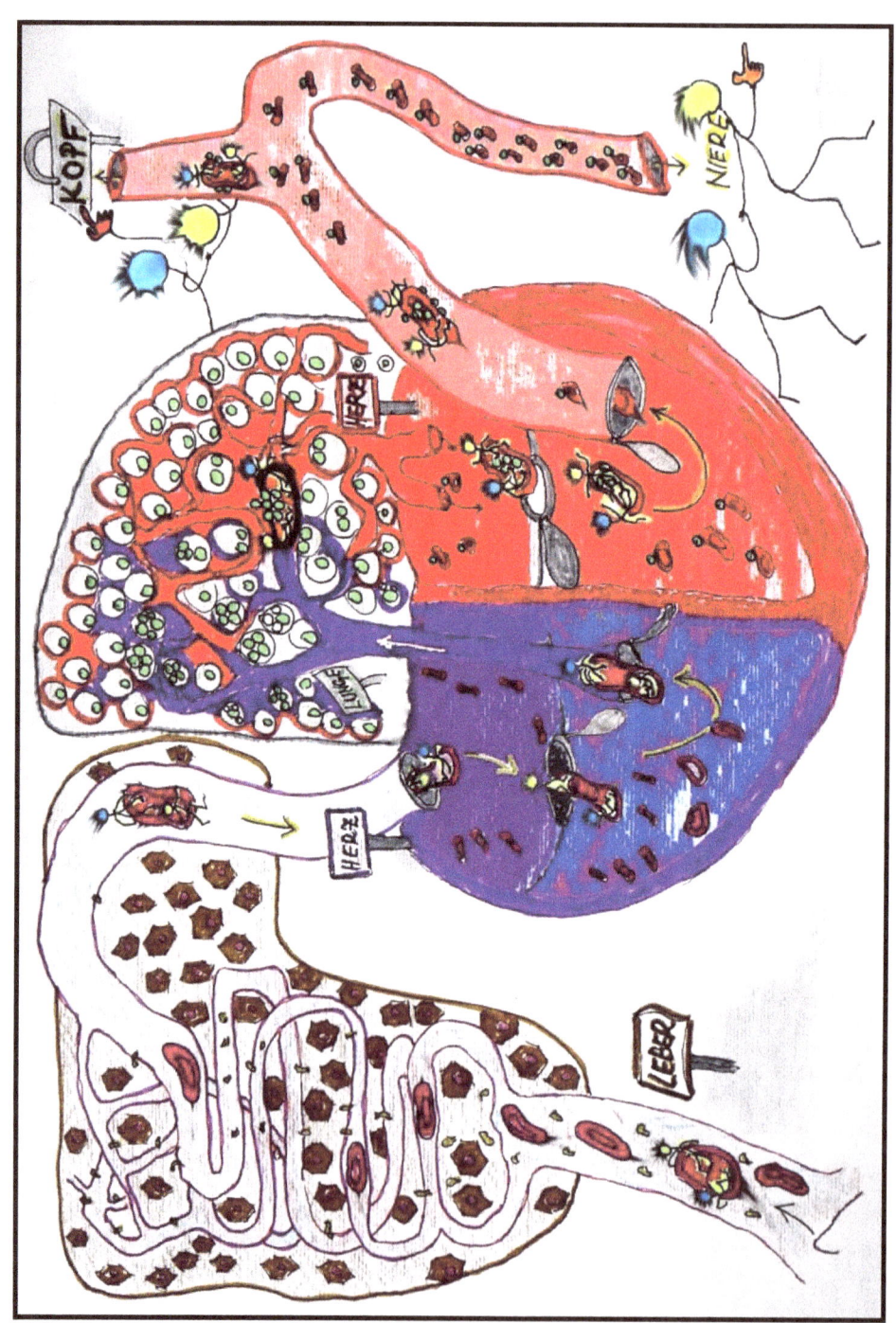

A fawn-colored city sign appears in front of them. ***"Leber-Liver"*** is written on it.

"Look," shouts **Chlory**, "that's where the noodle mush is being processed." Indeed, this is where all the mush silently disappears in deep cracks, gone forever. **Sod** and **Chlory** steer their boat into the middle of the blood stream, because they don't want to get off in the liver.

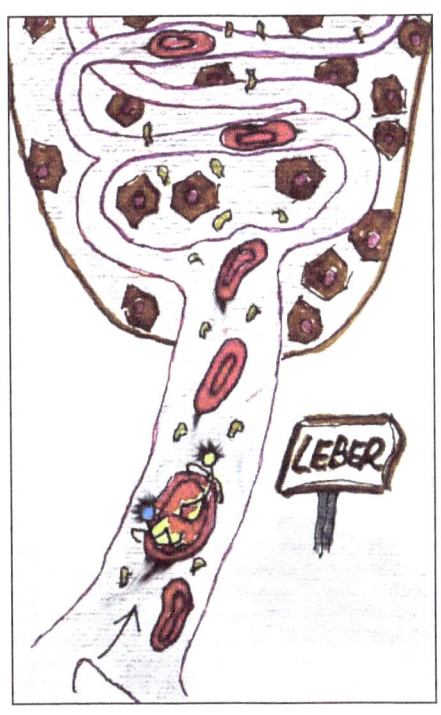

After a few minutes, they come to a purple town sign. *"Herz-Heart"* is written on it. Suddenly, the smooth ride ends and their boat is tipped into a purple room. As soon as they arrive there, a gate opens on the opposite side, through which their boat elegantly whizzes.

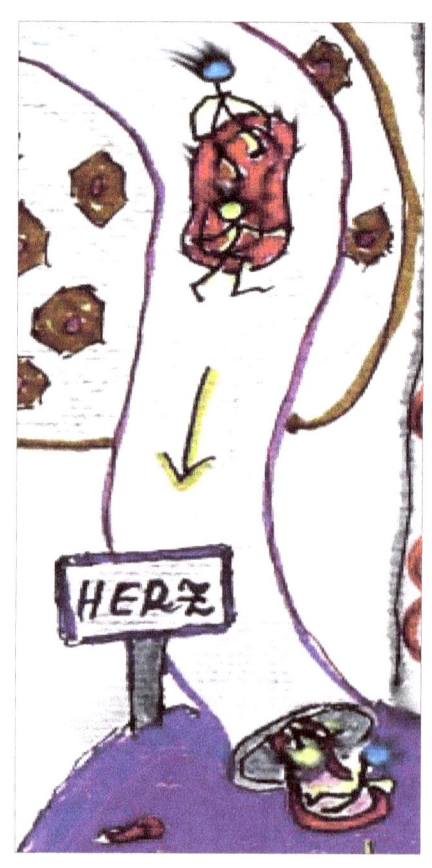

They enter a spacious cave and are whirled around wildly. A violent stream of blood hits them and on they go, almost in the opposite direction.

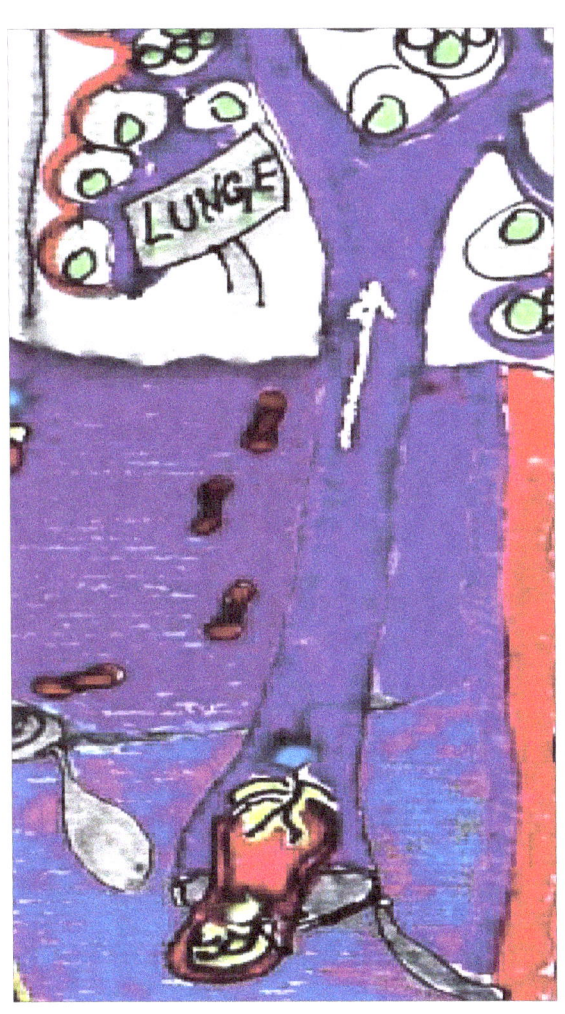

A door opens - plop - and off they go, right into a tunnel. There, on the left, they find a town sign again. It says *"Lunge-Lung"* in toxic green.

Now the bloodstream becomes much calmer. It branches out into many small channels that seek their own routes through the rough terrain. It becomes narrower and narrower. Through the thin walls, they perceive violent gusts of wind.

"Moritz is breathing," **Sod** whispers.

While **Sod** and **Chlory** stow the balls in the footwell of the boat, they leave the narrow channel, which finally opens into a wide stream.

All around them are boats loaded with green oxygen balls.

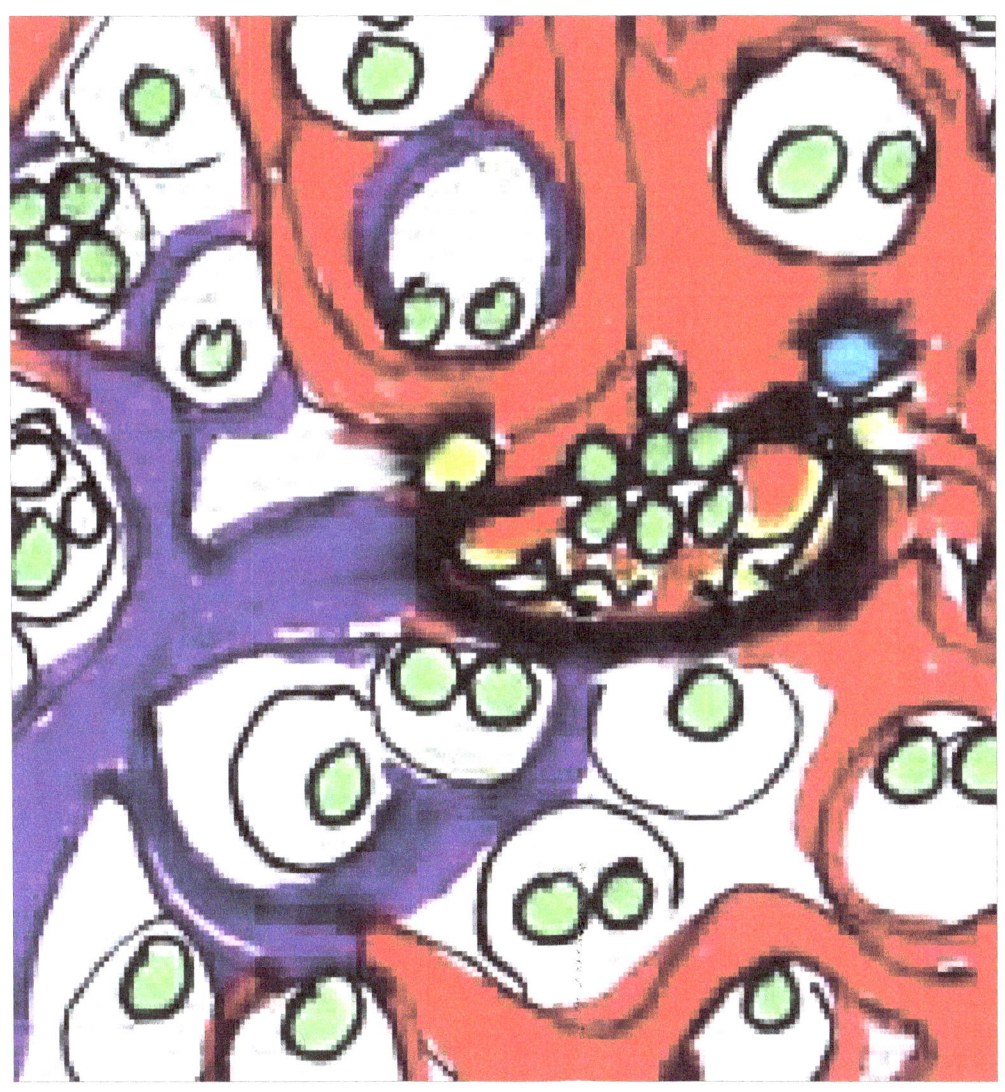

It's a sound that he first heard inside the chamois, way back when they were experiencing such miracles as smelling, hearing, and seeing. When their boat almost gets stuck in a particularly narrow channel, something unexpected happens. As if by magic, little green balls pop out of the wall and roll into their boat. **Sod** picks up one of these balls.

What a surprise!

The green balls are oxygen.

Again they pass a town sign with the same inscription as before, *"Herz-Heart"*, but this time in bright red.

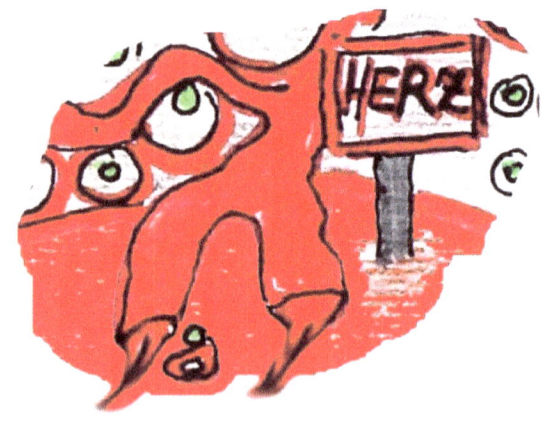

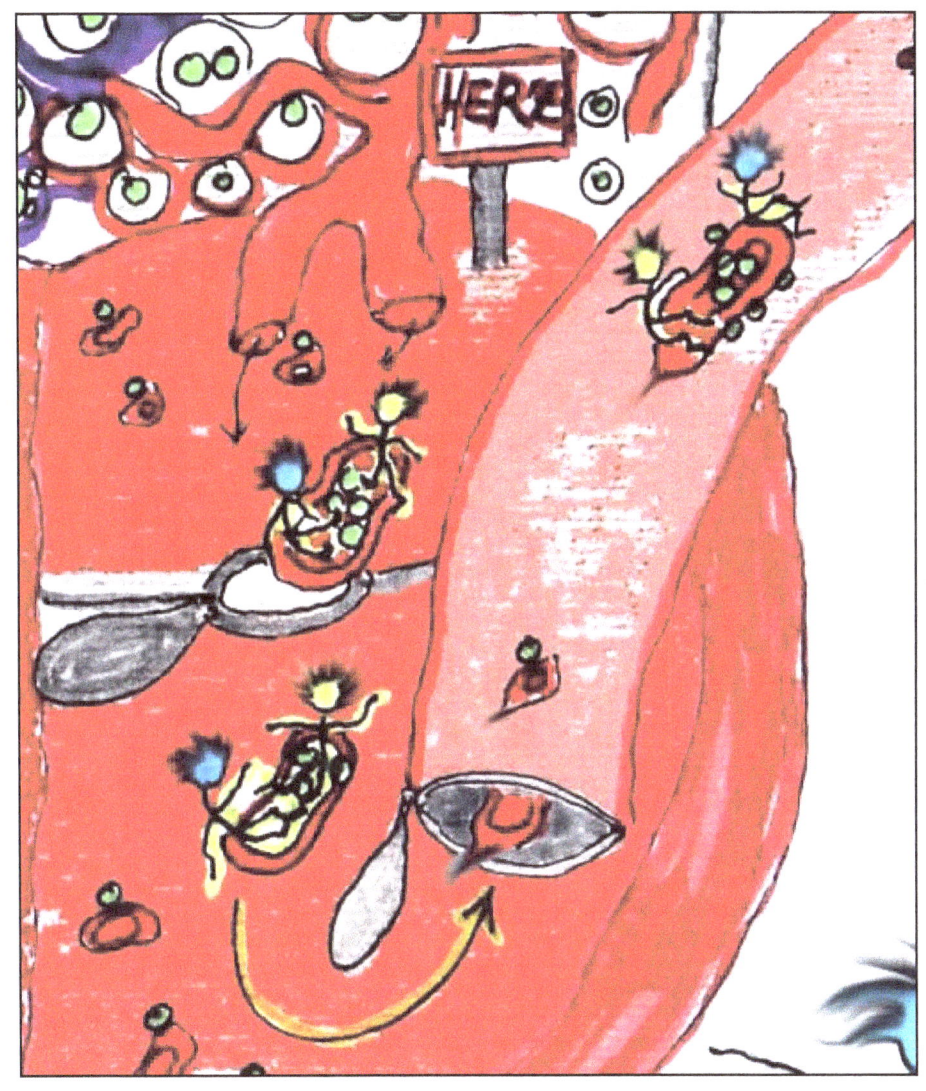

Smoothly, they enter a fiery red cave connected by a wing door to another large cave. Their boat is whirled around and they have to keep their hands busy to avoid losing any oxygen balls.

Finally, with a loud bang, a gate opens in front of them, through which their boat slips. They end up in a wide stream that jerks them forward.

"I'm getting really sick of this jerking," **Chlory** complains. "There's a junction coming up, maybe it'll get better then," **Sod** tries to comfort her. They turn left into a smaller side arm. It's still jerking, but not as violently.

Sod and Chlory travel through the head

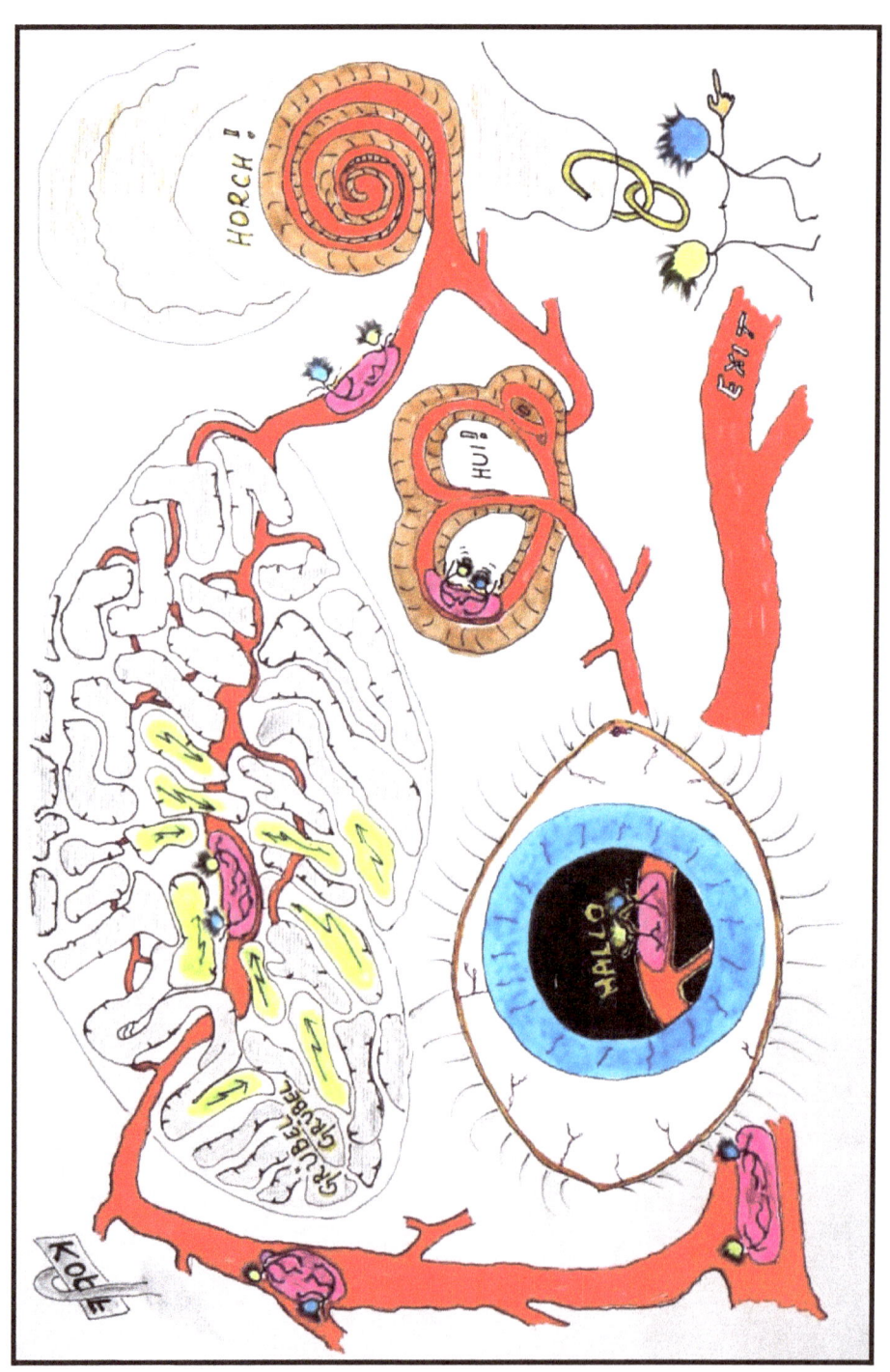

A mousy town sign pops up right in front of them.

*"**Kopf-Head**"* is written on it.

Sod and **Chlory** can't get out of their amazement.

"Now we're probably in Moritz's head, because our boat has been going uphill in a constant stream of blood," **Sod** muses.

All around them is pitch dark night. But suddenly a beam of light hits them. **Chlory** straightens up in the boat and waves excitedly. **Sod** follows her lead.

"If I'm not mistaken, we're just passing through Moritz's eye and peeking out into his world!"

They see Moritz's parents just sitting in front of their plates at dinner. *"Hello!"* the two call out as if from the same mouth.

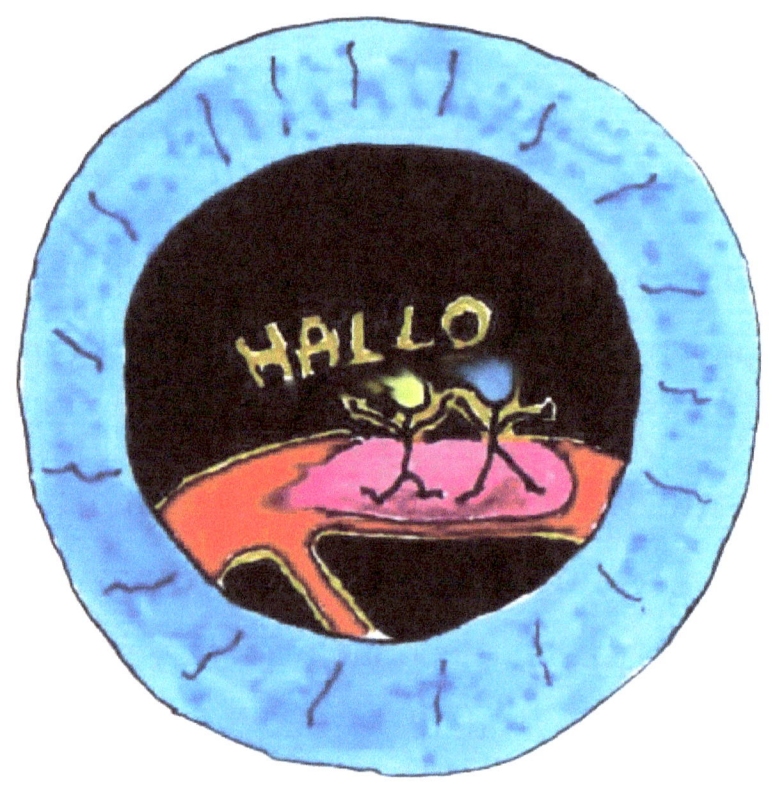

Hardly having left the eye, a wild roller coaster ride follows. Their boat travels through a labyrinth of narrow corridors, going up and down at breakneck speed. But a second later, it's pitch dark again. Only the gentle pounding of the waves on the outside of the boat can be heard.

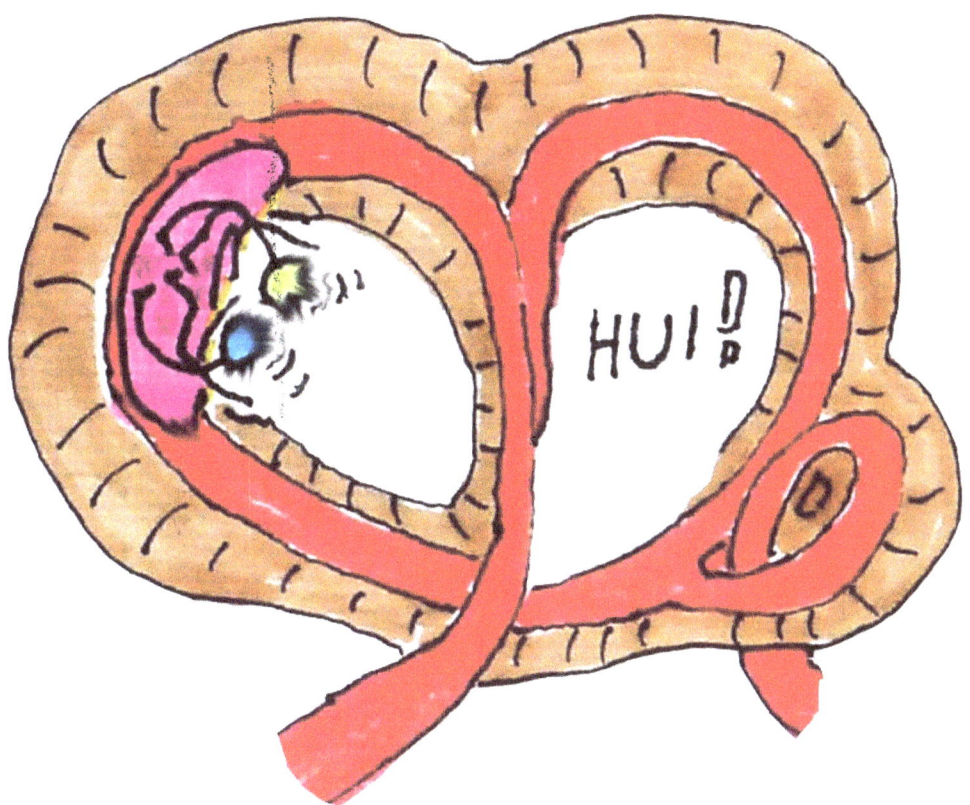

"*Hui*, everything is rotating in my crystal head," moans **Chlory** anxiously.

"We have to keep our balance so that we don't capsize," **Sod** says in a firm voice, waving his arms.

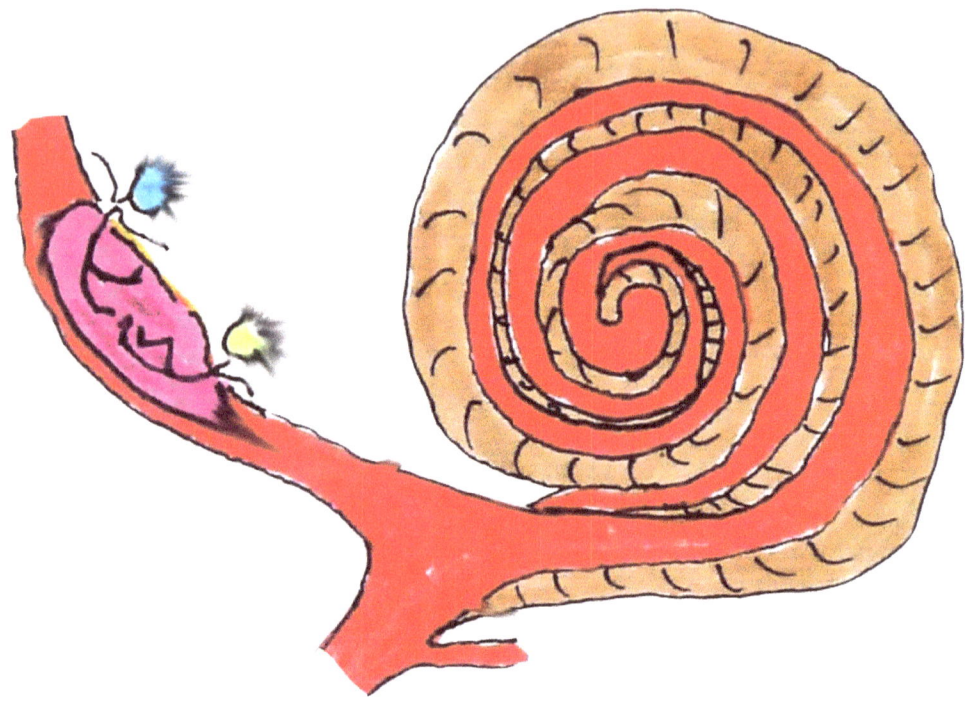

Finally, this hellish ride is over and they get back into calmer waters.

But the calm doesn't last long.

Their boat skids around a tight bend and then they ascend a spiral staircase, as if in a snail shell, all the way to the top. As soon as they reach the top, they hear voices.

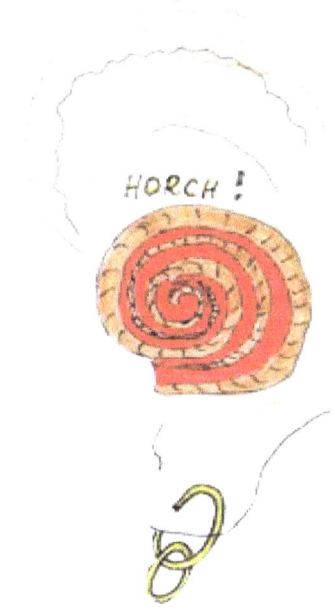

"Moritz, would you like another chocolate pudding for dessert or is your belly already too full?"
"That's mother's voice," **Chlory** whispers.

"Sure, chocolate pudding always has room in my belly."
"That's Moritz's voice," **Sod** whispers excitedly.

But in the next moment, they are already descending, down the spiral staircase. The voices dwindle.

Sod and **Chlory** lean back, exhausted.

The ride continues.

Everything around them is pitch black. Suddenly, bright flashes of light appear everywhere, eerily illuminating their surroundings.

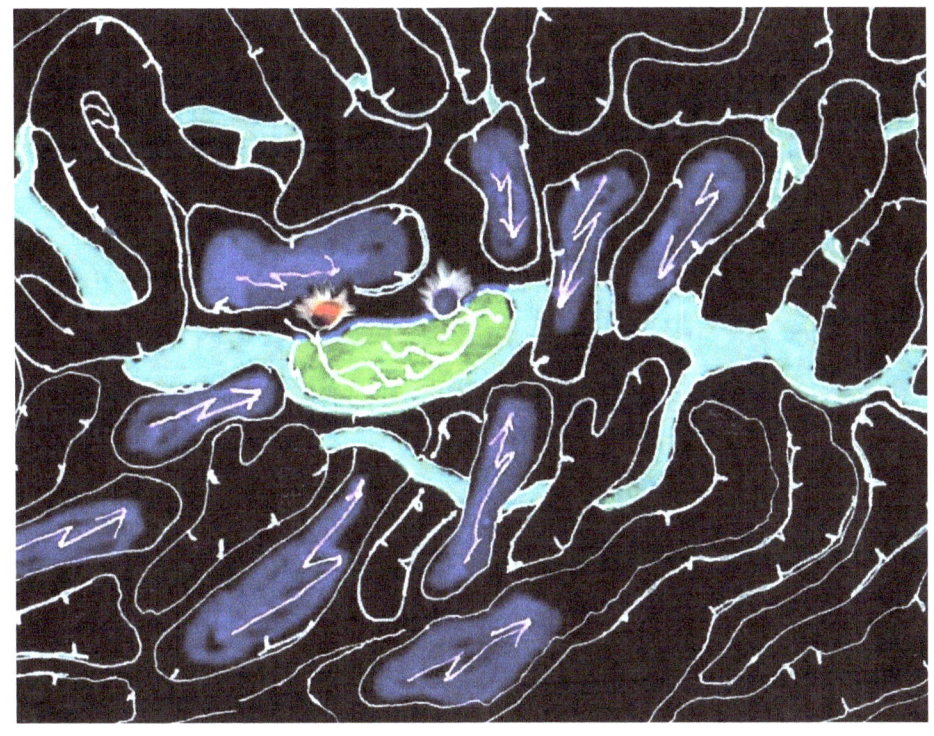

Suddenly, **Sod** says in a solemn voice:

"I think I know what this thunderstorm means. Moritz is thinking about the chocolate pudding! The flashes of lightning are the thoughts whizzing through his head."

"I hope we get out of this thunderstorm soon, I feel pretty scary," **Chlory** croaks in an anxious voice.

Sod takes her in his arms comfortingly.

"Just be patient," he says, "we'll eventually get out of here again."

Patience the two of them have, for they have infinite time! They are crystals, after all, and crystals are known to live forever and ever.

Sod and Chlory travel through spleen, kidney and bladder into the open

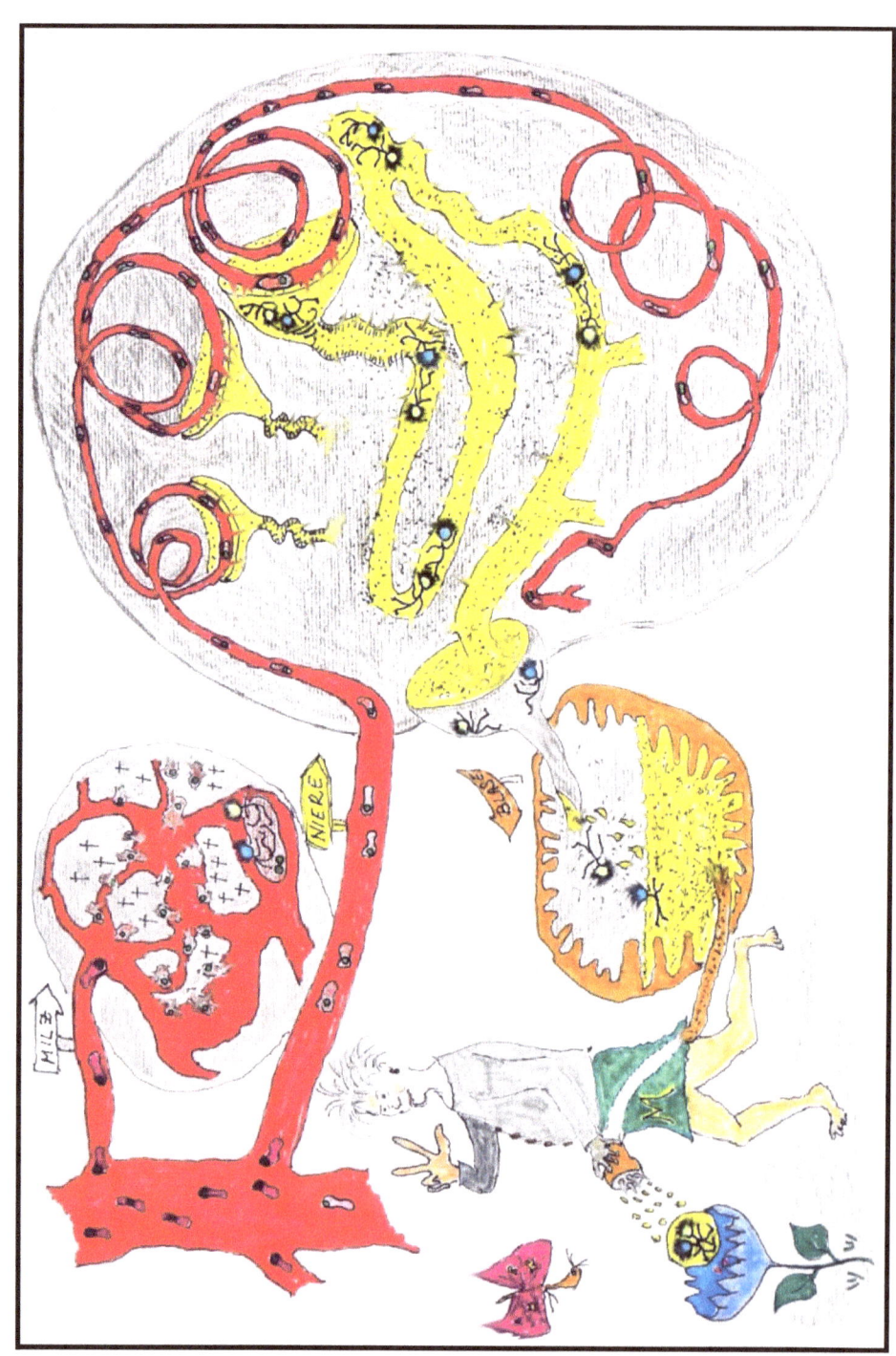

As suddenly as the thunderstorm came upon them, so suddenly it was gone again. The river, where their boat was now, became wider again and their journey calmer.

Eventually, they turned left into a side arm.

A signpost, white as snow, appears.

*"**Milz - Spleen**"* is written on it.

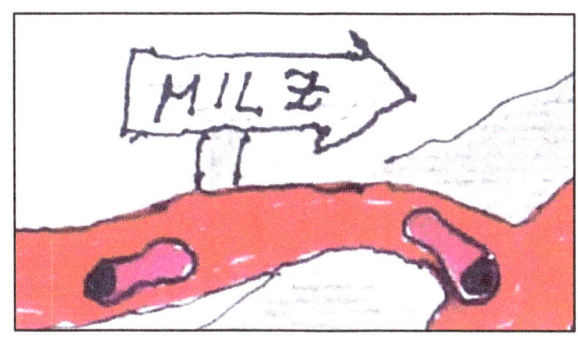

Shortly after, they notice a lot of boats that the bloodstream has obviously washed up on shore. They are riddled with holes and cracks, and just about to fall apart. "It's a real boat graveyard," **Chlory** marvels.

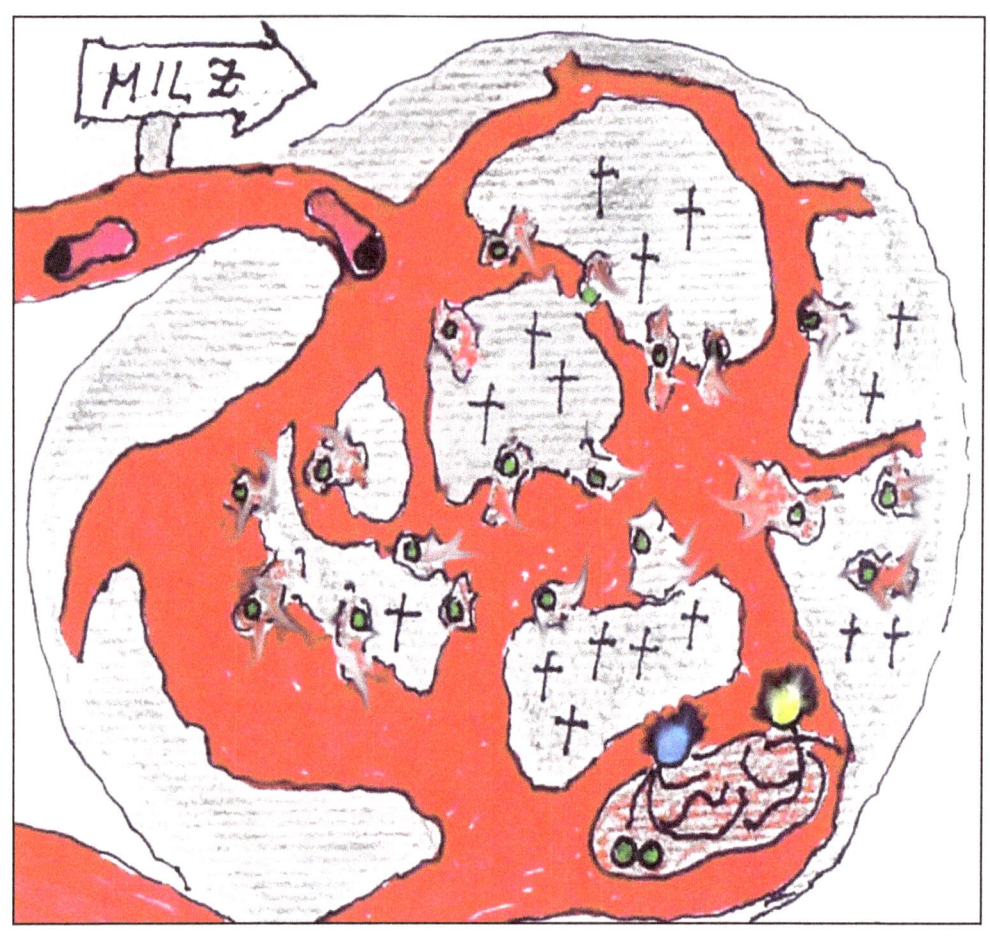

"I'm glad our boat is still in such good shape," **Sod** says almost proudly. Relieved, they leave the desolate boat graveyard behind them.

After some time, they come to a junction. Two side arms branch off to the left and right. Their boat whirls around as if it can't decide where it wants to go. Then, with a swing, it turns into the left side branch. After a while, a squeaky yellow signpost appears.

"**Niere - Kidney**" is written on it.

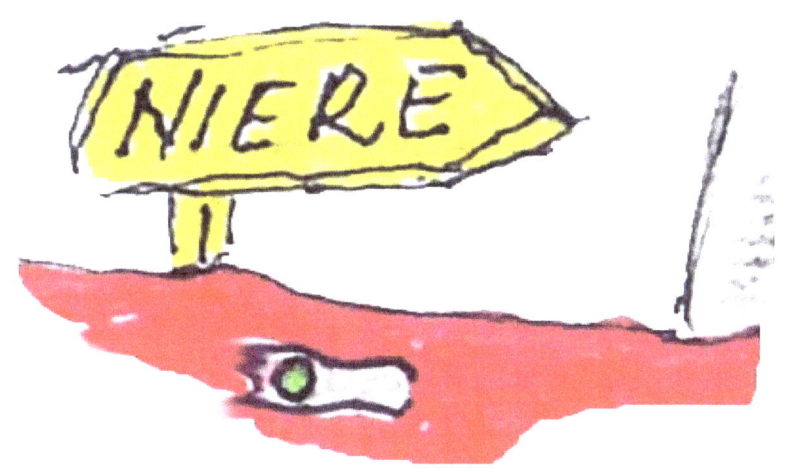

"Let's be surprised," says **Sod** and holds **Chlory** tightly so that she doesn't fall out of the boat.

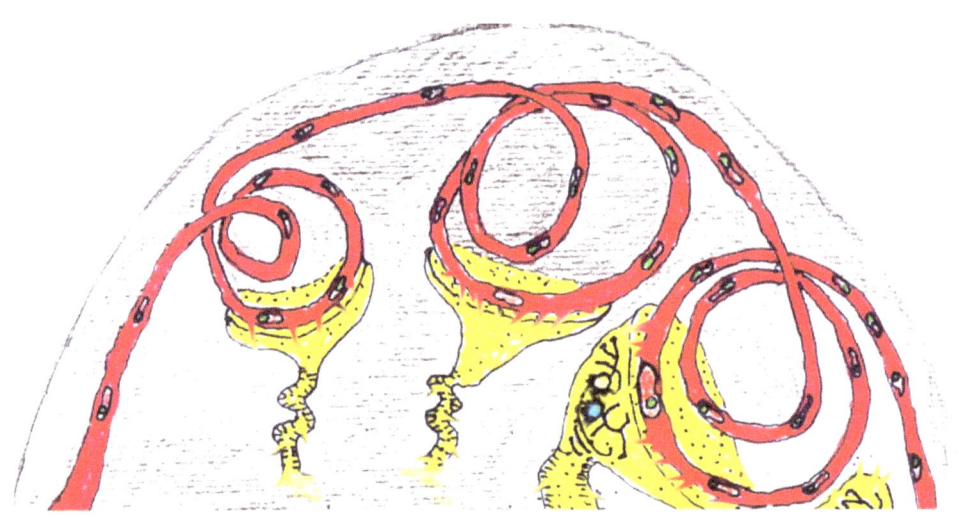

Yes, such danger is imminent!

In breakneck loops, they whiz through the bloodstream in their red speedster. It is getting so narrow that their boat almost touches the slippery side walls. Darkness prevails everywhere around them. Only sometimes there is a glimpse of light, just for a few moments.

Chlory has an idea.

"Don't you think we should try to get out as soon as it gets lighter?"

"We'll do that," **Sod** exclaims, "I'm already sick from this hellish ride."

So they whiz through the darkness one last time in their roller coaster until it suddenly brightens.

"Ready, set, go!" **Sod** shouts and courageously jumps out of the boat. **Chlory** clings to his heels. With a loud splash, they land in a clear, *yellow* lake.

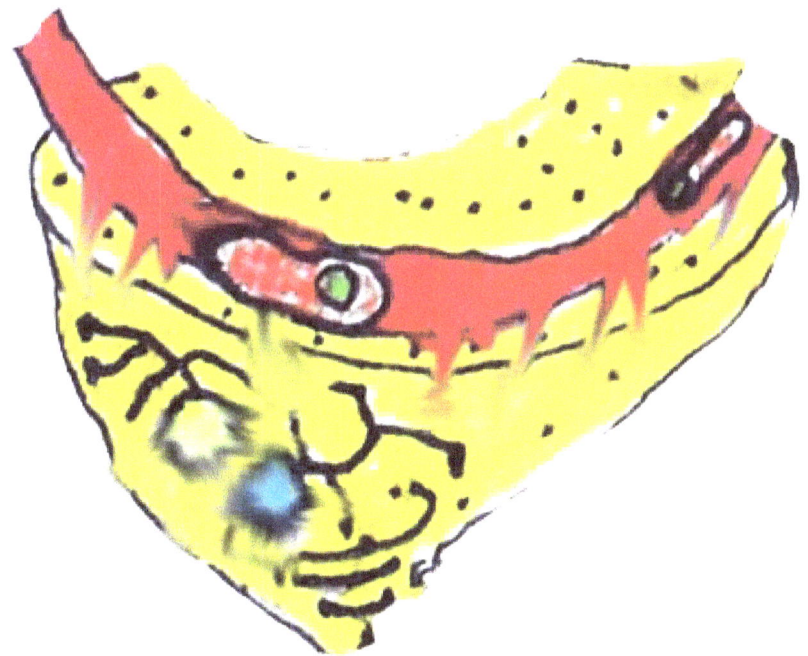

Far and wide, there is no boat to be seen.

"That's not blood," **Chlory** notes, "more like water. It reminds me of the sea. Let's just let ourselves drift with the current and wait to see what comes."

But the calm is deceptive.

As if by magic, **Sod** and **Chlory** are suddenly caught up in a vortex that pulls them down and only lets them go again in a channel. The walls of the channel are not smooth but overgrown.

"Looks like the seaweed at the bottom of the ocean," **Chlory** says, observing how here and there some sugar crystals washed into the channel with them and gradually disappear into this dense mesh.

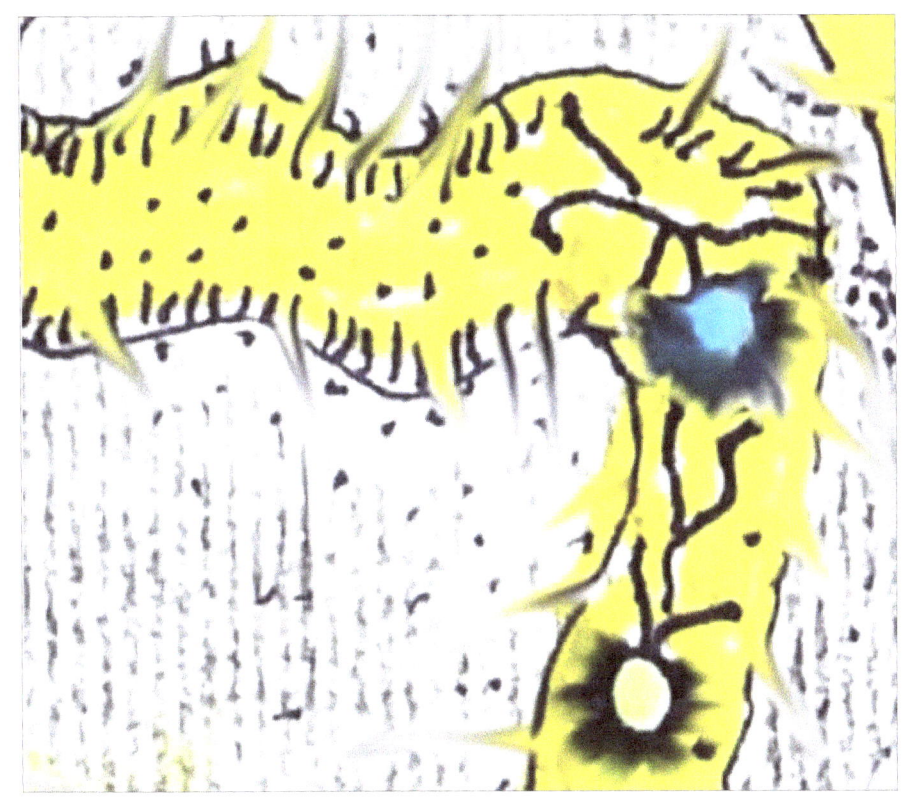

"Let's just drift downstream," **Sod** suggests, following the countless meanderings of the canal. Quite surprisingly, the canal suddenly leads them into the depths. After a sharp hairpin bend, however, they immediately head straight up again. As they swim by, **Sod** notices that the channel has tiny holes here and there. He notes with some dismay that some of their travelling companions are disappearing into these holes.

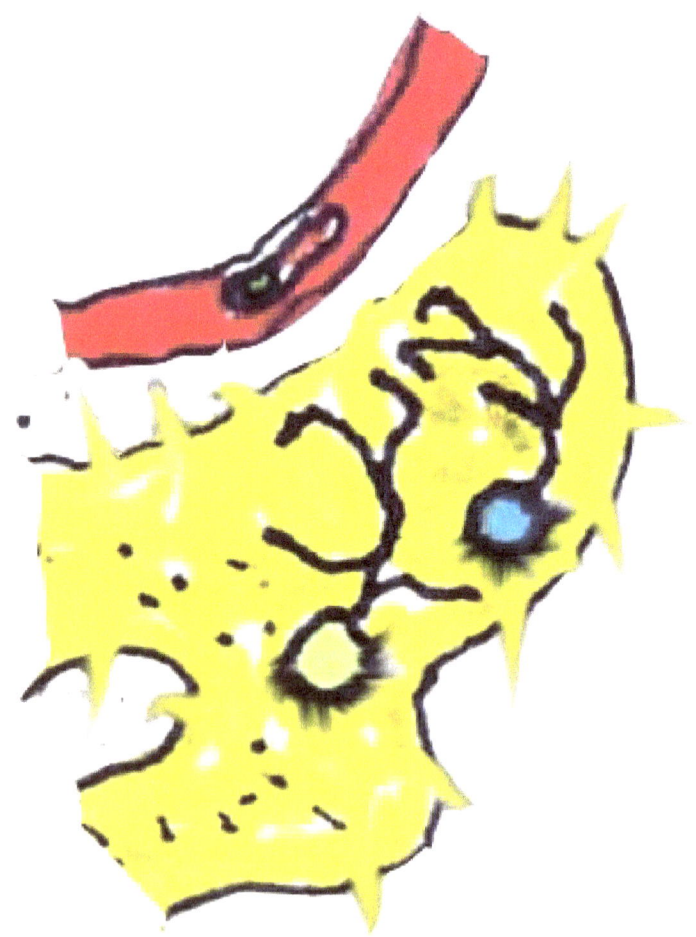

"If we stay in the middle of the channel, the holes can't swallow us," **Sod** whispers, pushing himself off the wall. **Chlory** stays close to him.

After a few turns, a long straight section of the channel follows. The two breathe a sigh of relief. They are now heading downstream in calm waters. Now and then, small rivulets flow from the sides into their river bed.

"Do you think it smells a little weird here," **Chlory** says.

"I think we're surrounded by all kinds of filth," **Sod** replies, pinching his nose. I am slowly getting glad when we have this hellish ride behind us and can finally get out again."

"Out of the kidney?" asks **Chlory** quietly.

"I mean, all the way out, namely out of Moritz. I would really love to see the sun again.

But yet they have to be a little patient. Surrounded by a nasty broth, the two are dumped into a large lake that is drained through a thick pipe at the very bottom.

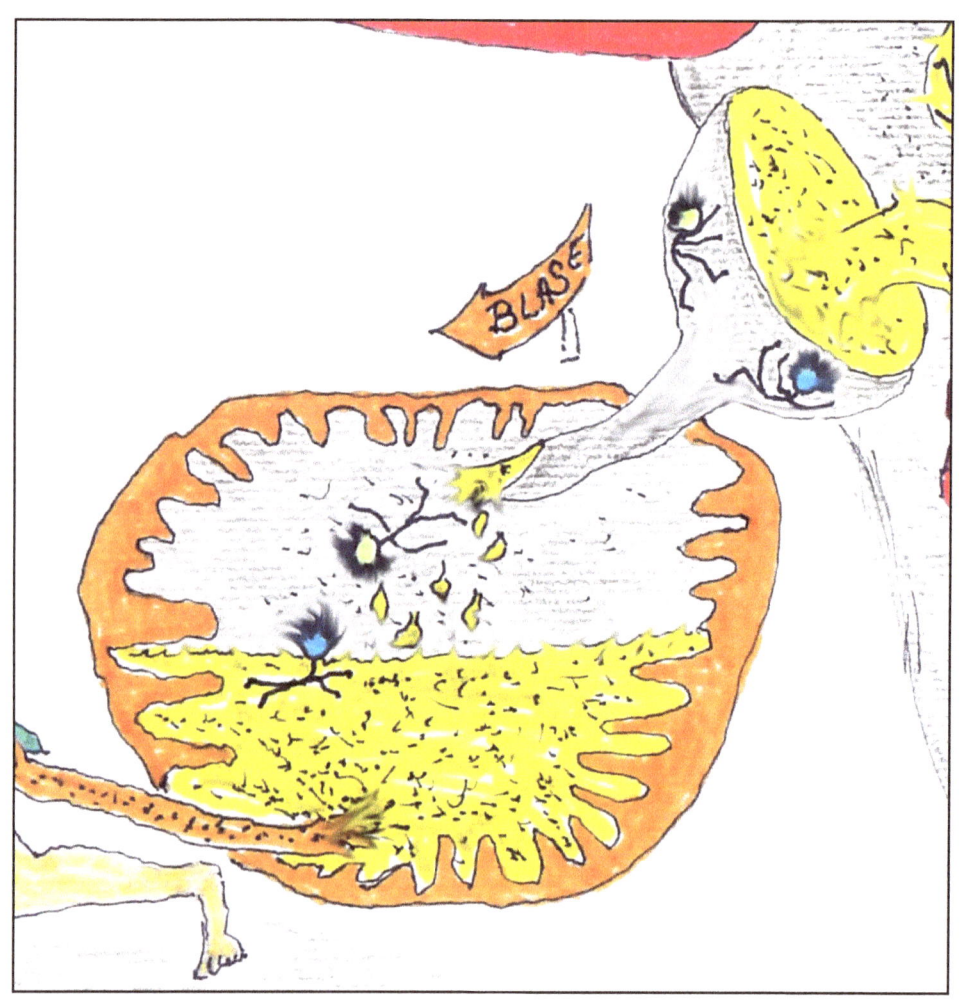

"Do you also feel the strong undertow?" asks **Chlory**.

"Yes, it's pulling us down," **Sod** says thoughtfully.

Indeed!

The two are sucked into the drainage pipe by a violent vortex and, after a rapid ride, are spat out at the open end.

They can just perceive the signpost ***"Blase - Bladder"*** as they whiz by, before they land in the water after a free fall through airy heights.

"Are we in the ocean now?" asks **Chlory** as they resurface.

"No, I don't think so," **Sod** replies, "I neither see the moon nor the stars. Besides, the sea isn't that dirty," he says, wiping the mess off his crystal head.

It is very quiet around them.

"Let's just wait and see what happens," **Chlory** suggests.

"We'll see the sun again someday," **Sod** comforts her. "If I'm not mistaken, we're still stuck inside Moritz. We're swimming in a subterranean pool where all kinds of trash has accumulated. But I believe that soon the moment will come and we will be free again."

"Actually, it's quite wonderful for us," **Chlory** *says softly to* **Sod**. *"The two of us, you and I, a long time ago, received some miraculous properties of human beings in the intestines of a magic chamois. Yet we have remained a salt crystal, traveling through the world without ever passing away. Humans are born and eventually they die. But we live on, in the human being, in the animal, in the plant."*

While the two of them are in close embrace, Moritz has gone to bed and is asleep.

The next morning the sun wakes him up. He jumps out of bed and his first walk is into the garden.

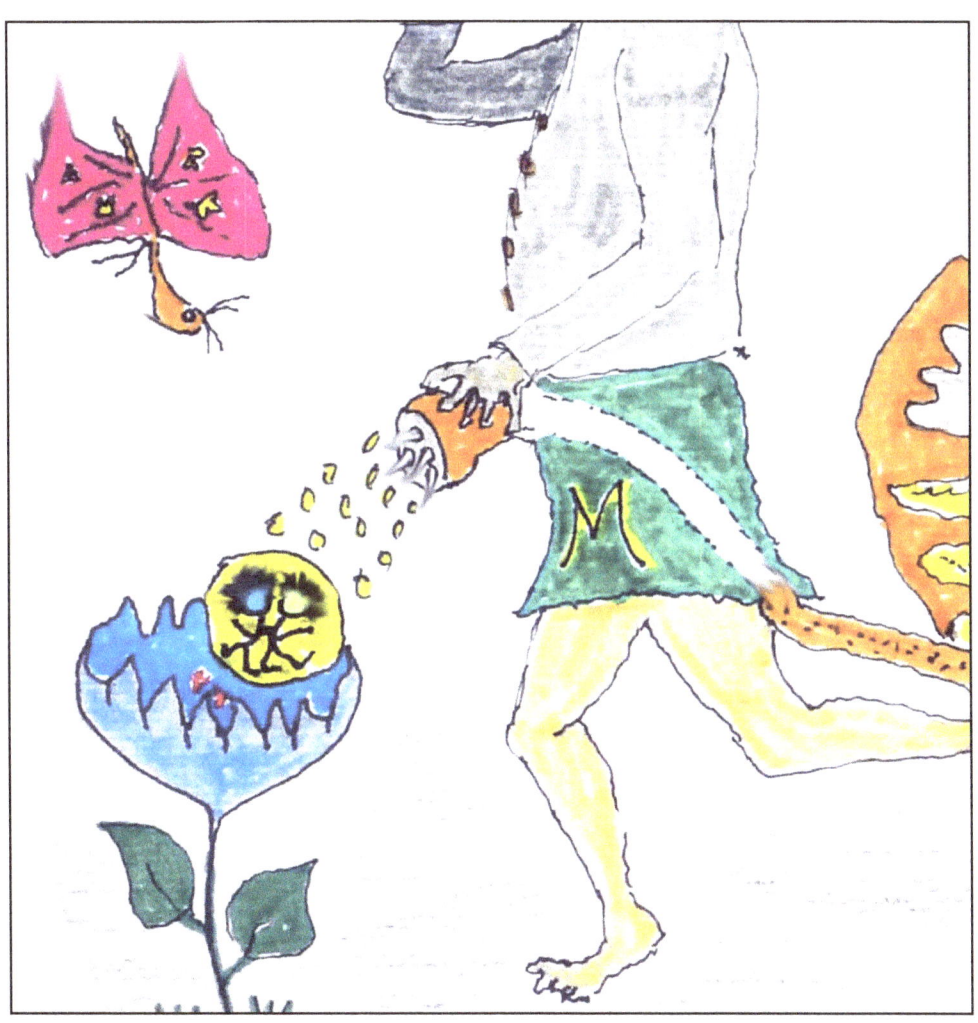

This brings life to the smelly pond where **Sod** and **Chlory** had spent the night. The calm waters begin to flow and in a gush of water, the two are pulled into a dark tunnel they hadn't even noticed before. After a frantic ride, they suddenly see light at the end of the tunnel. Shortly after, they are washed ashore by a violent jet of water.

"Finally sunshine again, exclaims **Chlory** excitedly, Moritz has flushed us out into Nature!"

Relieved, the two sit, nestled close together, in a drop of water, at the very top of a bellflower's calyx.

"**Sod**, after this exciting journey, we need some rest, don't you think?" says **Chlory**, laughing so happily that her crystal teeth just sparkle and glisten in the sun. "But the next adventure is already waiting for us," says **Sod**, pointing to a butterfly about to settle on the bellflower for some refreshment from the drop of water.

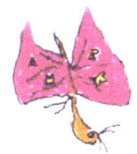

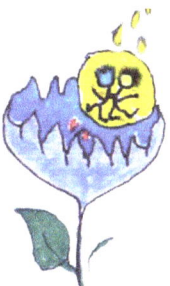

"I've always wanted to fly with you around the world in a butterfly," **Chlory** says exuberantly, rubbing her crystal head affectionately against **Sod's** shoulder.

Right then, the butterfly's antenna dives into the drop of water and brings **Sod** and **Chlory** on board.

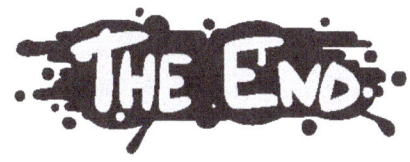

Another Children's book (paperback and e-book)

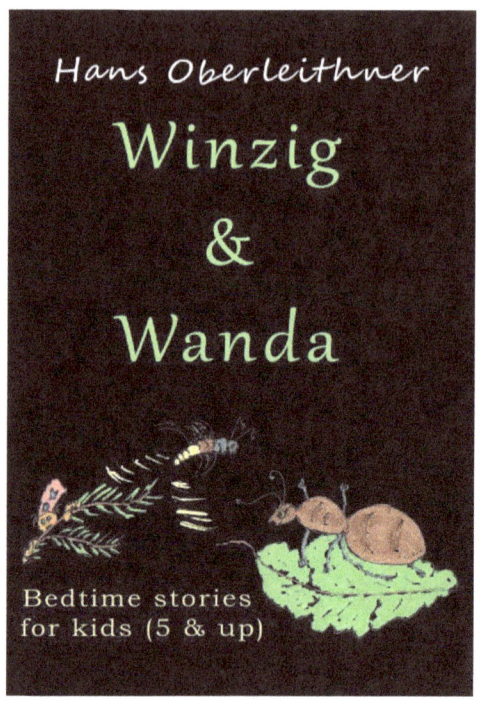

Winzig and his wife *Wanda* live in a snail house. In the wild garlic forest they escape a dangerous attack by a jay. On a cuckoo they sail through the air. In an earth tunnel they bump into a mole cricket. They travel to far-away dwarf cities visiting their grandkids and ... even learn the *Ant Language*.

Seven cheerful bedtime stories for kids (5 & up)

www.ingramcontent.com/pod-product-compliance
Lightning Source LLC
Chambersburg PA
CBHW060002230526
45472CB00008B/1904